Palliative Care for People with Learning Disabilities

Other titles available in the Palliative Care series:

Fundamental Aspects of Palliative Care Nursing by Robert Becker and Richard Gamlin

Palliative Care for the Child with Malignant Disease edited by the West Midlands Paediatric Macmillan Team

Palliative Care for the Primary Care Team by Eileen Palmer and John Howarth

Why is it so Difficult to Die? by Brian Nyatanga

Palliative Care for People with Learning Disabilities

edited by
Sue Read

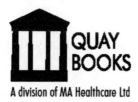
QUAY
BOOKS
A division of MA Healthcare Ltd

Quay Books Division, MA Healthcare Ltd, St Jude's Church, Dulwich Road, London SE24 0PB

British Library Cataloguing-in-Publication Data
A catalogue record is available for this book

© MA Healthcare Limited 2006
ISBN 1 85642 218 6

Printed in Malta by Gutenberg Press, Gudja Road, Tarxien PLA19, Malta

CONTENTS

LIST OF CONTRIBUTORS

Charlotte L Clarke is Professor of Nursing Practice Development Research and Associate Dean (Research), School of Health, Community and Education Studies, Northumbria University, UK

Jacqueline Furniss is Care Manager, Choices Housing Association, North Staffordshire, UK

Lynn Gibson is Senior Physiotherapist, Northgate Hospital, Morpeth, Northumberland, UK, and a community paediatric physiotherapist

Edward Lindop is Senior Lecturer, School of Nursing and Midwifery, Keele University, UK

Dorothy Matthews was appointed to the UK's first permanent Macmillan nurse post for palliative care in learning disabilities, Northgate & Prudhoe NHS Trust, UK, in 2004

Linda S McEnhill is a palliative care social worker, social work practice teacher and master practitioner in NLP. She works for the NNPCPLD and is also part-time lecturer at St.Christopher's Hospice, London, UK

Regina McQuillan trained in palliative medicine in London and Cardiff. She was appointed Palliative Medicine Consultant at St Francis Hospice and Beaumont Hospital, Dublin, Ireland, in 1996

Heather Morris is Project Coordinator, MENCAP Sharing Caring Project, Stoke, UK

Michelle Persaud is Nurse Consultant (Dual Diagnosis), Southern Derbyshire Community Mental Health Trust, UK

Siri Persaud is a former community nurse (learning disabilities) and now works in a national secure forensic service for women

Sue Read is Lecturer, School of Nursing and Midwifery, Keele University, Staffordshire, UK

Claud Regnard is Consultant in Palliative Care Medicine, St Oswald's Hospice, Northgate & Prudhoe NHS Trust and Newcastle City Hospitals Trust, UK

Karen Ryan is a graduate of the Faculty of Medicine of University College Cork, Ireland. She was awarded a Health Research Board Health Services Fellowship and is currently undertaking the two-year research project as part of an MD thesis

John Swinton is Professor in Practical Theology and Pastoral Care School of Divinity, History and Philosophy, University of Aberdeen School of Divinity with Religious Studies, Scotland, UK

Stuart Todd is Senior Research Fellow, Welsh Centre for Learning Disabilities, Department of Psychological Medicine, Cardiff University, Wales, UK

FOREWORD

So strong are the joint taboos of death and disability that it frequently comes as a huge surprise to organisations and carers when one of their service users becomes terminally ill and dies; or dies suddenly, as is more often the case. Services may in hindsight realise that the signs and symptoms of the illness were there for some time, but unseen until the end. Often, this becomes the source of deep regret which, when defended against, does not facilitate the type of changes necessary to ensure that 'history' does not repeat itself. This book is written for services, policy-makers, students and individuals who either proactively wish to avoid such a situation or, having experienced it, wish never to do so again. Its importance, therefore, cannot be underestimated.

It is a huge privilege to be asked to write the foreword for this book as it forms something of a landmark in an almost barren landscape. As the editor's preface says, it is a 'first' in bringing together the emerging knowledge held by a small group of academics and practitioners in this developing field. It is again testimony to the power of these taboos that, although authors such as Sinason, Hollins, Cathcart and Oswin laid the foundations for our thinking about the impact of death on people with learning disabilities (albeit from a bereavement perspective), it has taken some decades for others such as Tuffrey and Blackman to arise and build upon that knowledge-base. In the interim period, we have learned that people with learning disabilities not only grieve but also die. No longer hidden away in long-stay hospitals, people with learning disabilities and their dying have become public issues. Yet it is clear that the taboos are alive and well and consequently mainstream services are singularly unprepared to meet the often complex needs of this client group at the end of their lives.

It is therefore particularly appropriate that Persaud's chapter should open this book by recontextualising us with a historical perspective on the lives of people with learning disabilities over the last century. After reading this chapter, one will have a better grasp of why British people with learning disabilities have been so dangerously disconnected from primary healthcare services, and why there has been until now little pressure on these services to adapt to accommodate their needs. Persaud's chapter is followed by Todd's deeply thoughtful sociological analysis of the connection between death and learning disability — the consequence of which is that 'the deaths of people with learning disabilities appear to be deaths that have been too readily overlooked and infrequently discussed'. This will not be the case for any longer due to Todd's unique contribution.

Furniss' chapter roots us back into the lived experience of people with learning disabilities who are dying and maps out for us the professional networks that are necessary to engage if we are to come close to approximating a 'good death' for those in our care. With the luxury of time or forethought, Furniss demonstrates that this is an entirely achievable goal.

The issues of palliative pain and symptom control are often very complex and none potentially more so than in the care of people with learning disabilities who may have multiple co-morbidities, complex pre-existing drug regimes and communication difficulties. The chapter by Regnard *et al* is therefore vital reading. The wisdom of this chapter is borne out of joint working across the disciplines of palliative care and learning disability. Its gift to this book is the establishment of the idea that such complex needs can be assessed (by baseline recording) and addressed in a proactive way, which reduces distress and thereby enables other non-physical needs to be explored and a reasonable quality of life to be achieved right to the end.

The learning-disability nurse may well be the person who has known the patient consistently over many years; however, this is a role that is not well-understood in primary health care and especially within secondary care such as specialist palliative care. Persaud's chapter is therefore very useful in making clear the unique contribution that this professional can make to the dying person with a learning disability, and again borne out of years of experience it has much to teach us.

Increasingly, the decision-making processes of the medical profession are coming under intense scrutiny. The pendulum has swung far from seeing the doctor as 'the expert' to seeing him or her as but one of a number of professionals, each with their own unique expertise and valid opinions. This may well be the case and it is an important tension to hold given the very real power which historically the medical profession has held in the lives of people with learning disabilities. That being said, the stringent ethical underpinning of medical training makes doctors uniquely suited to navigating the moral maze that often surrounds the learning-disabled person at the end of their lives. Unless one has direct experience of palliative care, it may not be at first obvious that such thorny dilemmas are everyday — the arguments over whether or not to treat, and quality over quantity of life.

Read's chapters on communication and counselling will facilitate the adaptation of practice for the psychosocial professionals within the palliative-care team. Amazingly, their dying, if dealt with sensitively, may be the opportunity for the person with learning disabilities to deal with a number of unresolved issues. Read's practice-based wisdom makes this more likely.

Perhaps one of the most neglected areas of care for people with learning disabilities is that of spiritual care. Swinton's chapter highlights some of the reasons why this is the case, and why many religious institutions have been either unwelcoming or severely limited in their understanding of the person with a learning disability's ability to express both spiritual need and spiritual competence. At the end of life, for many, spiritual issues and questions of ultimate meaning become of prime importance. There is no reason for us to suspect that this should be any different for the learning-disabled person. Swinton's chapter enables us to reflect on these issues and equips us to begin working on both facilitating and meeting these needs.

McEnhill's chapter takes a look at the development of the modern hospice movement and its neglect of people with learning disabilities within it. However, its value-base means that the adaptation need not be as huge as one at first may think. The keys elements of listening to the individual and of working in a multidisciplinary team are explored. It is the individual whose story is told here — and who has the wisdom to offer, rather than the institution itself.

The final chapter is given over to the topic of research in palliative care and learning disability. This is of vital importance given the dearth of reliable information that we have on these topics currently. Lindop's chapter enables us to think through the sensitivities related to ethical research in this area and also points to areas that require further attention. It is a fitting close to a book that, hopefully, will spur practitioners and academics on to think new thoughts and test them out for the benefit of people with learning disabilities at the end of their lives.

It has been said that statistics are 'people with the tears removed'. This could also be said of many academic books, no matter what their area of focus. However, it cannot be said of this book. Not only does this book contribute a wealth of new knowledge, but it does so by interspersing the theoretical thinking — which is vitally important — with casework and the wisdom of seasoned practitioners. Much more importantly, it does so by projecting the voices of those whose experience teaches us much about our frailty as practitioners, but also about the importance of striving to try, tentatively, to get it, if not right, then better. My wish is that we are able to hear clearly and succinctly within its pages the echoes of these learning-disabled people who have so willingly shared their wisdom at the end of their lives, and that we might learn from them and become 'good enough' carers for those who follow them.

Linda S McEnhill
Coordinator NNPCPLD
December 2005

PREFACE

This book is probably the first of many textbooks that will focus on the potential issues involved when learning disability and palliative care combine to produce complex situations in the palliative-care context. It will be an important text, and will help to raise the profile of this neglected area. I intended to generate a text that was informative, easily accessible, interesting and useful to the range of professionals involved in delivering and providing palliative care to people with learning disabilities. It may not contain all the solutions to the complex dilemmas involved, but it does highlight the potential challenges we face and offer strategies to support and promote good palliative-care practice for this client population.

Dr Sue Read
Keele University, UK
December 2005

ACKNOWLEDGEMENTS

My grateful thanks to my friends and colleagues, who have expressed interest, shared the challenges and offered unconditional support throughout this journey. To Robin and Chris, who both patiently put up with many hours of me being secreted away in my study — thank you for your tolerance and understanding.

I would particularly like to thank my fellow contributors for their time and effort in contributing to this book. These experts in the field are all very busy people, who all care passionately about their respective interests. It has been a fascinating, tiring, exciting and adventurous journey.

Finally, this book is dedicated to all those people with learning disabilities who have let us into their lives and taught us so much about life's most painful lesson: death and dying. The lessons, sadly, continue.

Dr Sue Read

Historical perspectives — care for people with learning disabilities over the past century

Michelle Persaud

Care for people with learning disabilities has changed beyond recognition over the past century. It is essential to our understanding of the present, and indeed the future, to look back at the delivery of health services for people with learning disabilities, and to examine the principles on which their care was based. This chapter gives an overview of how people were cared for from 1913 in large hospitals; the effect of institutionalisation on them; and how they were viewed by society as a whole. It will address the effect of this transition from institutional hospital care to community-based services on their ability to access the services that others take for granted, particularly palliative-care services. It will also address the impact of the new theories that changed the way we perceive groups that society regards as 'different', thereby shedding light on the ways in which people with learning disabilities became marginalised.

Overview

In the late 1960s, there were roughly 60,000 people with learning disabilities living in hospitals in the UK, and many more living in the community (Lindsey, 1998: 71). Government policy began to concentrate on moving these people away from long-stay institutions to community provisions. The 1972 White Paper *Better Services for the Mentally Handicapped* recognised the negative impact of institutionalisation and segregation on people's lives, and that people with learning disabilities didn't necessarily require an institutional-care environment. This resulted in a national move to re-house people in 'ordinary' communities with the ambitious target of reducing the number of beds to 5000 by 1997.

In that year, New Labour continued the policy of the previous Conservative government by maintaining the programme of closing down long-stay institutions. They also acknowledged, as had many others in the field, that 'the move from large institutions to small size accommodation does not automatically ensure that the type of care provided will be any less "institutional"' (Brown and Smith, 1992: xvi). In the hope of addressing the inequalities faced by learning-disabled people, the Government published *Signposts for Success* (Lindsey, 1998), which turned out to be a landmark document, detailing good practice for commissioners and providers of healthcare services for people with learning disabilities. The main theme of the document is captured in the opening words: 'the National Health Service was founded on the principle that good quality health services should be available to all' (Boateng in Lindsey, 1998: 1).

As social-policy directives continue the decommissioning of large institutions, people with learning disabilities are using community services more than ever before. This includes health services that will be required to take a full part in maintaining the health of individuals who may have greater needs than most. This is especially true of the last people to move from large institutions, as they tend to have the most complex health needs (Hayward and Kerr, 1998).

Good quality lies in the nature and scope of services available — and quality of care is paramount in the delivery of services to people with learning disabilities. It is difficult, however, to measure quality of care when the person being cared for is unable to speak for themselves, and when services have changed so drastically over the past two decades. The changes are both political and social: political, in the shift of emphasis for health care to be provided within an internal market; social, in the sense of policy development embracing a philosophy of human services that are provided within the community. Critics of the move away from hospitals would argue that the agenda, far from being a humanitarian one, was more cynically grounded in fiscal policy, rather than social or health policy. Current service provision for people with learning disabilities looks very different now to the way it did in the 1960s, when the ideas and principles of a theory called 'normalisation' were just emerging in the UK healthcare system.

In 1913, the Mental Deficiency Act was introduced. It prescribed paternalistic care and, more importantly, protection for people who had acquired the label 'mentally defective'. It established a 'Board of Control' that was directly responsible to the House of Commons via the Home Secretary. The Board was in the powerful position of 'assisting to breed out the hereditary transmission of mental defect by preventing the propagation of a degenerate stock' (Potts and Fido, 1991: 140). The Act defined four main categories of defect:

- **Idiots** — persons unable to guard themselves against common physical dangers.
- **Imbeciles** — persons whose mental defectiveness does not amount to idiocy, but who are incapable of managing themselves or, in the case of children, could not be taught to do so.
- **Feeble minded** — persons whose mental defectiveness does not amount to imbecility but who are in need of care, supervision and control for their own protection, or, in the case of children, could not benefit from instruction within a school.
- **Moral defectives** — persons whose mental defectiveness is coupled with strong vicious or criminal propensities that need controlling for the protection of others.

Fuelled by the calls of people such as Mary Dendy in the 1890s that children classified as 'mentally defective' should be 'detained for the whole of their lives as the only way to stem the great evil tide of feeble-mindedness in our country', there was demand for the creation of new public institutions culminating in two thousand such places being available by 1914 (Potts and Fido, 1991: 10).

Life in these institutions (or 'colonies', as they were also known) was grim. Rules and regulations were strictly designed to ensure the smooth and efficient running of the institution: '[they] did not allow for individual self-expression, nor did they permit some basic human rights.

The institution controlled everything, including contact with parents, relatives and the world outside' (Potts and Fido, 1991: 57). It is no wonder that society came to accept the fate of learning-disabled people as being one of segregation and hospitalisation. Locked away from mainstream life, these people rapidly came to be seen as 'deviant' or 'subnormal'. 'You never went out for anything because [they] did everything in the hospital' (Cooper, 1997: 24), 'everything' including all health care and treatment. Life was confined to the institution. Health care and health screening amounted to a very cursory examination on admission by a consultant psychiatrist. He (the doctors tended to be male) would check the ears and chest. The usual type of entry to records would be 'chest field appears clear. No obvious illness or infestation'. This 'examination' would be repeated anually with the resulting record entries stating 'remains the same' (Beacock, 2001: 56). As late as 1980, there were still nurses training for the title 'Registered Nurse — Mental Subnormality', and the care was provided within a medical, paternalistic context.

In the 1970s, a new theory emerged, which was to become internationally influential in human services: 'normalisation' (Flynn and Nitsch, 1980: 3). As with any new theory, it generated much debate and gained as many critics as exponents. Even now, the debate is far from finished, although it is universally accepted that the theory is built on the principles of quality of life and services. Bank-Mikkelsen (1969), who was head of the Danish Mental Retardation Service, was instrumental in having the concept of normalisation written into Danish law in 1959. He postulated that normalisation should mean 'letting the mentally retarded obtain an existence as close to the normal as possible' (Wolfensberger, 1980: 75). This marked the beginning of the normalisation debate in an international context (even though it still belonged primarily to 'mental retardation' [learning disability] services). In a keynote address to a 1977 conference of rehabilitation educators, Wolfensburger discussed, in a general way, the 'role that service agencies play in the twin and opposed processes of deviancy, devaluation and normalisation' (Flynn and Nitsch, 1980: 4).

Whereas Wolfensberger applies these principles universally for all 'deviant people', Bengt Nirje (1969) described normalisation in relation to mental retardation services. Although Wolfensberger is often seen as the 'father' of normalisation by some, and as the person who finally took the concept and illuminated it by others, all three authors — Bank-Mikkelsen, Wolfensberger and Bengt Nirje — are what commentators would call 'classical definers' of 'normalisation', and all deserve recognition.

What is 'normalisation'?

Since Wolfensberger introduced it into North America in the late 1960s, the theory of normalisation has evolved into a systematic and guiding principle for the design and delivery of services for all 'devalued' people, but mainly people who are learning-disabled. Wolfensberger's version has had the most impact in the UK than its predecessors. He writes:

> *Normalisation implies as much as possible the use of culturally valued means in order to enable, establish and/or maintain valued social roles for people.*
>
> Wolfensberger and Tullman (1989: 29)

It is assumed from this principle that human services therefore have a major role in the improvement of people's valued roles, and in defending them if devalued.

Critics of normalisation are keen to point out that even if the principles are based on providing 'normalised' services, interpretations vary. Some professionals incorrectly assume that normalisation means that the person, as opposed to the service, is to be 'normalised' (whatever that may mean). But normalisation is 'not something that is done to a person. It is a principle for designing and delivering the services a person needs' (O'Brien, 1981: 26). Conversely, Walker and Walker (1998) assert that this is one of the main arguments against the philosophy (as they call it). They state that even with 'normal' provision, there could be inadequacies and inappropriateness for varying service users. What becomes clear is that any philosophy, principle or concept is always subject to misinterpretation, whatever its author's intention.

Highly conscious of this, Wolfensberger, in his later work, discarded 'normalisation' in favour of 'social role valorisation', and in his book about the subject introduced the concept as being born out of normalisation. He called it a 'high-order concept for structuring human services' (Wolfensberger, 1992: 1). Like Goffman before him, he understood that the social identity of people who were 'mentally retarded' (learning-disabled) was 'stigmatised' and that these people were (and, arguably, still are) given a different or lesser service or existence compared with the 'normal' or 'ordinary' person.

Goffman (1963: 11) identified the person who was stigmatised as being someone who was different. The stigma isn't necessarily a physical sign on the body but something 'applied more to disgrace itself than to the bodily evidence of it'. He says that, collectively, humans have rules and norms of behaviour that are acceptable: something he calls 'social intercourse'. When we are alike and in the presence of each other (he argues), these rules, which govern social intercourse, help us anticipate others. However, when a stranger arrives, we tend to assess his or her social identity (rather than social status) by appearances. The implication for people with learning disabilities is profound, especially when there are also physical attributes that vary from the 'norm'.

Bogdan *et al* (1982) argue that human beings transmit stereotypes and characteristics of devalued or deviant people largely through what is called 'the unconscious association of social symbols or images'. There are abundant examples of these images in popular culture: one need think only of, say, Captain Hook or Frankenstein's monster.

Wolfensberger (1992: 11) has suggested that society uses negative social roles to identify a devalued person as:

- Other — ie. alien, different.
- Non-human — seen as human once but no longer: ie. a senile or comatose person.
- Menace — object of menace or dread, or threatening in nature.
- Object of ridicule — the butt of jokes or amusement.
- Object of pity — afflicted, felt sorry for.
- Burden of charity — society has a duty of care but only at the most basic subsistence level.
- Child — two forms: the eternal child who never matured to competent adult; and the adult who is having a 'second childhood' — a person with dementia, for instance.
- Diseased organism — the person in the role of the sick or diseased organism requiring therapy or treatment, usually dispensed by medical personnel in medical surroundings (hospitals, clinics).

Particularly pertinent in the field of learning disability are the last two categories, which, arguably, are the way many people with learning disabilities are still viewed, consciously or subconsciously, even in the twenty-first century.

In 1999, the Department of Health (DoH) carried out a review of the quality of services for people with learning disabilities, which resulted in a report entitled *Facing the Facts* (DoH, 1999a). It exposed many deficiencies in health and social care for people with learning disabilities. Concurrently, the DoH completed a review of the Mental Health Act (1983), which concluded that subjecting people with learning disabilities to the provisions of the Act is wholly inappropriate. It also conceded that a citizen should only be subject to the authority of the legislation if he or she is suffering from a defined mental illness. Beacock (2001) argued that the Act is grounded in paternalism and protection, and that it is still used inappropriately in today's practice. Until new legislation is passed, in the form of a new Mental Health Act, people with a learning disability are still subject to being detained as being 'impaired', even in the absence of a defined mental illness. Because of the nature of learning disability, and the devalued social identity often ascribed to people who have it, helping learning-disabled people find or create valued roles (or enhance the valued roles they already have) becomes essential. Their right to equality of social opportunities and healthcare services is as strong as anybody else's.

Many studies about the health needs of people with learning disabilities show similar findings. Some specific conditions are more prevalent amongst this population than amongst the general population (Kerr *et al*, 1996). Identification and diagnosis of conditions and illnesses can be problematic because of difficulties in communication and understanding. Coupled with the fact that government health policy has traditionally excluded learning-disabled people from mainstream services, we now face a huge challenge in equipping services to meet the needs of these previously excluded people. This challenge falls into two halves: changing the culture and attitudes of providers; and giving services with the education and training needed to deal with learning-disabled people.

Cultural and attitudinal change

Beacock (2001: 62) asserts that people with learning disabilities have 'too little political influence to challenge the bastions of modern society and too small a voice to be heard above the clamour and din of competing interests at the healthcare table'. He develops this assertion by stating that when caring for people with learning disabilities and their health needs, 'it is not simply about health and illness; it is about valuing people who are not the same as you'. A policy of segregation has only exacerbated the negative perception and treatment of people with learning disabilities by society and, arguably, health services too.

Within a National Health Service that is already overstretched, there are many demands for resources and money. Attitudinal change also demands resources and money. It also takes time: it is a long and sometimes arduous process throughout systems that have been developed around institutional processes and routines, not necessarily people. Given that people with learning disabilities have the same illnesses as everyone else, but may also have communication and cognitive difficulties, these systems are challenged to help the person achieve the same health outcomes. Wilson and Haire (1990) describe the fact that health systems are 'reactive', meaning the individual needs to seek help in the first instance.

Before they even seek help, however, they must first be able to recognise that there is a problem. Kerr (1998), citing Kinnell (1987), asserts that because of communication difficulties, there will be under-reporting of symptoms of physical and mental illness within the learning-disabled population. Beacock (2001) agrees, arguing that mental illness, in particular, is under-reported. He goes on to claim that not only does lack of communication exacerbate under-reporting in this group, but also that the ability of carers and professionals to recognise symptoms needs to improve. He suggests that carers, both formal and informal, 'may well be inclined to interpret and treat behaviours, rather than symptoms'.

Matthews (2002) suggests that at the first interface of health service delivery, primary care, there is little knowledge about the needs of people with learning disabilities and how their health is compromised. He also suggests that there is an unrealistic expectation on the part of specialist services (learning disability) that primary care teams should provide health screening and surveillance for learning-disabled people. This would be in contrast to people in the rest of the population, who self-present and take responsibility for their own healthcare needs. What he argues is that specialist learning disability services (when given the appropriate training and tools to do the job) are highly effective in screening and surveillance, and that the outcomes for people with learning disability are significantly improved as a result. Tuffrey-Winje (2002), cited in Jones (2003), agrees, but strikes a cautionary note by pointing out that the timing of engagement of specialist services (palliative care, diabetes clinics, etc) is crucial, or people with learning disabilities may suffer delayed identification of life-threatening illnesses because of difficulties in diagnosis.

The challenge for change will undoubtedly be tested in the audit of health services, particularly primary care. Each strategic health authority must be able to prove the numbers of people with learning disabilities accessing services. This will require GPs routinely to record this information. Statistical data will indicate uptake rates for screening and surveillance services, but qualitative research will need to be carried out to identify how well services are achieving better healthcare outcomes for people with learning disabilities. One explicit policy directive from *Valuing People: a New Strategy for Learning Disability for the 21st Century* (DoH, 2001) is that every individual will have a health action plan. A person called a 'health facilitator' has a crucial role in developing this plan in partnership with the individual and primary health services. These plans are evolving documents that should reflect changes in the lifestyle and health needs of the individual, as necessary. The Government (via the Valuing People Support Team) has a responsibility to ensure that the targets are met within this policy initiative. Only audit will show if the rhetoric has been matched by reality.

Education and training

There is much work to do in this area. Education about the health needs of people with learning disabilities is required by the individuals themselves, by carers and by professionals in specialist and generic health services.

Learning-disabled people

People with learning disabilities have the same illnesses as everyone else, but evidence suggests that the uptake of general services is lower than that of the rest of the population. Not all people with learning disability know where to go for help, and even if they did, quite often the identification of an illness or health need in the first instance is absent. Many health and social services work jointly now to facilitate health promotion education programmes, which are proving successful in helping people to access the health care they need (see *Case Study 1.1: Harriet*):

Carers

Kerr (1998: 13) argues that people who are cared for are reliant on the skill and knowledge of others: not only must carers be knowledgeable in identifying signs and symptoms, they must also 'develop self-awareness in terms of personal ideology, values and prejudice to ensure the well-being of those in their care'. What he suggests is that theories such as normalisation are still misused because staff misinterpret them and jeopardise people's health by asserting that 'it was their choice' not to attend a GP appointment. It is clearly unacceptable within a care environment for this to happen and staff need to understand the context within which they care.

Another problem area is that people with learning disability are seen as just that: learning disabled. There are many horror stories in which a person has only been able to communicate pain or discomfort by behavioural distress and change. These changes have been attributed to the learning disability, whilst physical and health factors have been ignored, sometimes with tragic consequences. This ultimately leads to more mismanaged health care for people with learning disabilities, which Harriet's story (*Case Study 1.1:* Harriet) only illuminates.

Case Study 1.1: Harriet

Harriet was forty-nine years old and lived in a private residential home for people with learning disabilities. She attended a local-authority day centre. She always carried a bag with her that contained maternity sanitary towels. Harriet joined a 'healthy women's group' and told the facilitators that she was embarrassed by her incontinence. They referred her to a community nurse (learning disability) who assessed Harriet. She had very low self-esteem, lacked confidence, and missed opportunities for social engagement due to her worry of the incontinence. The staff where she lived had advised her to wear maternity pads to 'keep her womb warm'! The nurse excluded any physical cause for the incontinence (eg. infection) and found that she had stress incontinence. A programme was developed with Harriet to improve her pelvic floor muscle tone, and the nurse also carried out some basic education with the carers in the home. The programme lasted for six weeks, after which she was no longer incontinent. Harriet went on a holiday later in the year without bags and pads, and her confidence improved significantly. She now enjoys a very active social life and continues with her pelvic floor exercise routine.

Specialist services

'Specialist services' in this context means mainstream health services that specialise in specific areas of health need — eg. services for cancer, diabetes, coronary care, audiology, etc. These services are staffed with experts in the field. Many staff say they don't feel equipped to deal with people with learning disability; some feel afraid at the prospect of dealing with someone who may communicate differently from the 'norm'; and many have never had any formal education or training in the area. Although evidence suggests that services are recognising the right of people with learning disability to access mainstream services, they are still ambivalent about doing so. Styring (2003) reports that staff in mainstream services lack knowledge about the client group. She says it would be 'nonsensical to expect generic services to be able to meet their needs immediately' and that there is much work to be done in identifying these needs and going about achieving them.

Mainstream services and delivery

Because of the additional problems that people with learning disability face (communication and sensory deficits, mobility problems, etc), accessing services is quite often fraught with difficulties. Sometimes they may face fears and phobias about even *going* to a clinic or a surgery. Services need to recognise that a 'one size fits all' philosophy is inadequate. The Mental Health Foundation (1996) suggests that 'GPs should give attention to the atmosphere of their surgery for people with learning disabilities'. This should be true of all health environments, primary and secondary care. Services need to be flexible in their approach to individuals, offering longer appointments, first or last appointments of the day, and informal approaches to consultation. From my own personal experience as a community nurse (in 1995), I know that this is not always the case. I once accompanied a young woman for a health-screen check. The doctor insisted on wearing a white coat, even though it was explained to her that the woman was phobic about white coats and doctors. The result was that the young woman refused the health check and became extremely agitated. The doctor would not remove the coat because her attitude was that she was a doctor and that was her 'uniform'. She also explained, when challenged by the nurse, that she had to wear the coat because 'they [learning-disabled people] all have a certain smell that stays on your clothes'. The young woman refused to see that particular doctor again and subsequently became 'difficult' in her behaviour with other doctors. Clearly, this attitude is unacceptable and should be challenged, but it also shows that the legacy of the past still affects some professionals.

Commissioners

Commissioners need to be sensitive and knowledgeable when providing and purchasing services for this group of people. Service-led agreements should be comprehensive in the detail about extra services that learning-disabled people need. It is simply not appropriate to assume that if learning-disabled people are not mentioned in these important plans, this will mean inclusion — quite often, the reverse is true (ie. if they aren't mentioned, they *don't* get a service). Local boards for primary-care services should have representation in some form to enable the needs of people with learning disabilities to be considered in all planning.

Services have much to learn about working together in true partnership. There are many changes that can be made at a micro level, which would have a substantial impact on the care that people receive. Direct care workers should embrace the opportunity to make contact with other services to improve the experiences of people with learning disabilities who need specialist services, such as palliative care.

Research is vital. One (unpublished) study by Persaud (2001) illuminated the need for services to work together. There is evidence that supports the need for high-quality palliative care for people with learning disabilities, a need that is more important now than ever because people are living longer (Read, 1998; Tuffrey-Wijne, 1997; Keenan and McIntosh, 2000). We must meet the challenge of providing these services in timely, appropriate and accessible ways so that people with learning disability are treated as equal citizens.

Evidently, services that provide care must embrace quality of life and quality of care within their philosophies. The delivery must be evaluated to ensure that the stigmatisation ascribed in poor practice is constantly monitored and eradicated. Improvements should be made to ensure that vulnerable people are offered the socially valued opportunities that Wolfensberger and Nirje describe, and to which the rest of the population aspire.

Conclusion

It is clear from the historical perspective of learning disability care services that the nature and type of care received by people with learning disabilities has changed beyond all recognition from the days of the 1913 Mental Deficiency Act.

Goffman reminds us that consigning people to large anonymous institutions changed the nature of their existence and the way they were perceived by the 'outside world'. Pioneers of normalisation (which later became social role valorisation) have been successful in fuelling change in service design and delivery: they have made services think about the way staff attribute stigma to vulnerable people by the manner of their care for them. Their ultimate goal has been to attain better quality of life for learning-disabled people by challenging the notion that all such people should be treated in isolation in large institutions.

Contemporary policy reflects these changes, with many services attempting to meet the directives of community-based care for all people, regardless of need. To maintain quality and improvements, however, evaluation and research are essential. Services should embrace opportunities for practice innovation and look to colleagues in other fields of nursing to see what they can offer to improve what is currently available.

Research in the field of palliative care, for people with and without learning disability, is growing. Read (1998) describes the difficulties of people with learning disabilities when accessing services, and the measures required to overcome these difficulties. Persaud (2001) argues that services need to be more integrated to maximise resources, skills and labour. He proposes joint training and education for palliative care and learning disability services to improve the service-user experience. Both investigators urge services to work together and call for even more local and national research. Like the pioneers of normalisation, these researchers aim to examine, analyse and improve the quality of life and experiences of learning-disabled people. They have moved the agenda in palliative care forward by making the bold but necessary case for integrated, rather than separate, services.

There is much opportunity for joint- and partnership-working. Indeed, current policy demands that this will be the *modus operandi* for the future in all services for people. We need to collaborate and negotiate with our partners in health and social care to get a better deal for all people with learning disabilities.

References

Bank-Mikkelson (1969) Changing patterns in residential services for the mentally retarded. In: Flynn R, Nitsch K (eds) (1980) *Normalisation, Social Integration and Community Services.* Proed. Incorporated, USA

Beacock C (2001) Mental health and learning disabilities. In: Markwick A, Parrish A (eds) (2003). *Learning Disabilities: Themes and Perspectives.* Butterworth-Heinemann, Oxford

Boateng P (1998) Foreword. In: Lindsey M (1998) *Signposts for Success in Commissioning and Providing Health Services for People with Learning Disabilities.* DoH, Wetherby, Yorkshire

Bogdan R, Biklen D, Shapiro A, Spelkoman D (1982) The disabled: media's monster. *Soc Policy* **12**: 32–5

Brown H, Smith H (1992) *Normalisation: a Reader for the Nineties.* Routledge, London

Cooper M (1997) Mabel Cooper's life story. In: Atkinson D, Jackson M, Walmsley J (1997) *Forgotton Lives: Exploring the History of Learning Disability.* BILD Publications, UK

Department of Health and Social Security (1972) *Better Services for the Mentally Handicapped.* HMSO, London

DoH (1999a) *Facing the Facts: Learning Disability Services: a Policy Impact Study of Social and Health Services.* The Stationery Office, London

DoH (1999b) *Review of the Mental Health Act 1983: Report of the Expert Committee.* The Stationery Office, London

DoH (2001) *Valuing People: a New Strategy for Learning Disability for the 21st Century (Cm 5086).* The Stationery Office, London

Flynn R, Nitsch K (eds) (1980) *Normalisation, Social Integration and Community Services.* Proed. Incorporated, USA

Goffman E (1963) *Stigma: Notes on the Management of Spoiled Identity.* Penguin, Middlesex

Hayward B, Kerr M (1998) Accessing primary health care: pathways to care. In: Kerr M (ed) (1998) *Innovations in Health Care for People with Intellectual Disabilities.* Lisieux Hall Publications, Lancashire

HMSO (1913) *Mental Deficiency Act*. London

Jones A (2003) Palliative care and people with learning disabilities. *Learn Disabil Pract* **6**(7): 30–7

Kerr M, Fraser W, Felce D (1996) Primary healthcare needs for people with a learning disability. *Brit J Learn Disabil* **24**: 2–8

Kerr M (ed) (1998) *Innovations in Health Care for People with Intellectual Disabilities*. Lisieux Hall Publications, Lancashire

Kinnell D (1987) Community medical care for people with mental handicaps. *Ment Handicap* **15**: 146–50

Lindsey M (1998) *Signposts for Success in Commissioning and Providing Health Services for People with Learning Disabilities*. DoH, Wetherby, Yorkshire

Matthews D (2002) Learning disabilities: the need for better health care. *Nurs Stand* **16**(39): 40–1

Mental Health Foundation (MHF) (1996) *Building Expectations*. MHF, London

Nirje B (1969) The normalisation principle: implications and comments. *J Ment Subnorm* **16**: 62–70

O'Brien J (1981) *The Principle of Normalisation: a Foundation for Effective Services*. Campaign for Mental Handicap, London

Persaud S (2001) *Staff Perceptions about the Nature and Extent to which Palliative Care and Learning Disability Services Work Jointly in the Provision of High Quality Services for People with Learning Disabilities who are Terminally Ill*. Unpublished work for New Researchers Training Programme, The Trent Institute for Health Services Research

Potts M, Fido R (1991) *A Fit Person to be Removed: Personal Accounts of Life in a Mental Deficiency Institution*. Northcote House Publishers, Plymouth

Read S (1998) The palliative care needs of people with learning disabilities. *Int J Palliat Nurs* **4**(5): 246–51

Styring L (2003) Community care: opportunities, challenges and dilemmas. In: Markwick A, Parrish A (eds) (2003) *Learning Disabilities: Themes and Perspectives*. Butterworth-Heinemann, Oxford

Tuffrey-Winje (2002) Palliative care needs of people with intellectual disabilities: a case study. *Int J Palliat Nurs* **8**: 222–32

Walker A, Walker C (1998) Normalisation and 'normal' ageing: the social construction of dependency among older people with learning difficulties. *Disabil Soc* **13**(1): 125–42

Wilson D, Haire A (1990) Healthcare screening for people with mental handicap living in the community. *BMJ* **301**: 1379–80

Wolfensberger W, Glenn L (1975) *P.A.S.S. 3. Program Analysis of Service Systems — A Method for the Quantitative Evaluation of Human Services*. National Institute on Mental Retardation, Toronto

Wolfensberger W (1980) Research, empiricism and the principle of normalization. In: Flynn RJ, Nitsch KE (eds) *Normalization, Social Integration and Community services*. TX: Pro-Ed, Austin, Texas

Wolfensberger W, Tullman S (1989) A brief outline of the principle of normalisation. In: Brechin A, Walmsley J (eds) (1989) *Making Connections*. Hodder & Stoughton, London: 211–19

Wolfensberger W (1992) *A Brief Introduction to Social Role Valorisation as a High Order Concept for Structuring Human Services*. Revised edn. Syracuse University, NY: Training Institute for Human Service Planning, Leadership and Change Agents

CHAPTER 2

A troubled past and present — a history of death and disability

Stuart Todd

The modern learning-disability service and research communities pride themselves not only on having developed a commitment to providing as full and ordinary life as possible for people with learning disabilities, but also on maintaining this commitment 'from the cradle to the grave'. Yet when an individual's life is drawing to an end, our attention seems to wane, which I consider to be a hidden transition. Although there is a growing body of research that examines the impact of learning disability on life and living, what it means to die with a learning disability is unknown. There is very little research on where people die, or the quality of care they receive at the end of their lives.

Such reluctance does not merely result from death being a taboo subject in general, since there has been a greater willingness to talk about death over the past decade. Far from perceiving death as taboo, argues Walter (1991), we are rapidly becoming a 'death-obsessed' society, as popular and social-science examinations of the subject proliferate. As death is increasingly consigned to later life and secularisation spreads, the uncertainty about physical survival gives way to uncertainty about the meaning of survival and a growing anxiety about how one will die, rather than with what will happen after death.

Yet such shifts in attitude are not universal. Field, Hockney and Small (1997), for example, argue that, far from being the great leveller, our experience of death is shaped by the same forces that shape our lives, such as class, gender, ethnicity and age. And not all deaths seem to merit the same levels of attention or reflection (Lovell, 1997): the deaths of learning-disabled people are often too readily overlooked and infrequently discussed (Todd, 2002; McEnhill, 2004). Having a learning disability is just as likely to influence an individual's death as it did his or her life.

In this chapter, I will argue that professionals in the field of learning disabilities have collectively turned their backs on death to put a distance between past and present ideologies of care. In other words, death represents an unwelcome and disturbing reminder of previous social practices, when there was a tendency to perceive people with learning disabilities as 'as good as dead', or their lives as 'made-as-if-dead'. By contrast, current ideologies of care, which are based on the ideal of an ordinary and full life, unwittingly squeeze death out. The contemporary learning-disability community is increasingly concerned with the problems of living and, perhaps, of giving life back to those who were once 'made-dead'.

Although this philosophy may seem both desirable and humane, in banishing death from our day to day concerns we are undermining the value of the 'life' that is being given back. If death cannot figure within our community, what is the value of life being fought for? Todd (2002: 230) captures this irony when he writes: 'Death can only not count for those who have never lived or for those we wish to be lost from memory'.

My starting point is that we need to embrace death and find space for its discussion if our claim that we are committed to providing an 'ordinary' or 'valued' life is to be taken seriously. I will argue that death and learning disability are old, if forgotten, friends, and that we can use this link to face up to the challenges posed by death, and respond to them even more effectively and humanely than before.

Resisting mortality — the emergence of a new transition

One of the most remarkable changes for people with learning disabilities in the last century was their increasing longevity (Carter and Jancar, 1983; Patja, 2001). The life expectancy for the majority of these people has now come close to the norm. Although many people with more profound disabilities or with specific syndromes continue to have considerably shorter lives, the benefits of improved medical treatments and life conditions are clear for all groups of people with learning disabilities (Patja, 2001). Thus, for people with Down syndrome, life expectancy was nine years in 1929, eighteen years in 1963 (Collman and Stoller, 1963), and fifty-six years in the 1980s (Fryers, 1986). Patja (2001) reports that the relative risk of death is high for people under thirty with learning disabilities, but beyond this it comes close to the norm. Thus, the more people with learning disabilities who survive into late-early adulthood, the more likely it is that they will live into old age. Death has been pushed back, as it has been for the wider population.

However, these changes in mortality patterns have two main consequences that have not been fully considered by the learning-disability research community, nor by the service community: first, as people live longer, they are much more likely to die over a longer period of time; second, more people will enter the dying phase of their lives in some form of service setting.

Mortality studies are clearly beginning to show changes in the causes of death that come with increasing life expectancy. For younger people with learning disabilities, congenital abnormalities and infectious diseases are the most common causes of death (Similia, 1986); for older adults, the most common causes of death are cancer and respiratory and vascular diseases (Jancar *et al*, 1984). Indeed, deaths from cancer are rising from a relatively low baseline for this population, as they are increasingly exposed to cancer-related environmental factors and ageing (Patja, 2001). For the most part, mortality studies highlight improvements in the medical and social care of people with learning disabilities, and show that death is being increasingly postponed.

Ultimately, of course, death is inevitable, so these changes in mortality patterns have important implications for the nature of dying. As deaths from acute causes come to be superseded by chronic and degenerative diseases, death will become more expected rather than sudden, and dying may occur over a period of months rather than days. A new transition period, therefore, is taking place in the life-course of people with learning disabilities — that is, the transition period from living to dying, which few services seem adequately prepared for (Todd: in press). The pre-mortem implications of recent mortality research have barely been considered. Instead of recognition that dying and death should have great relevance within the field of learning disabilities, there is instead a reluctance to deal with it (Todd, 2002). I will now discuss the reasons for this.

Death and learning disabilities — troubled soul mates

Although death might seem a marginal concern in the modern learning-disability community, the dead, the dying and people with learning disabilities have long been seen as sharing a common fate, a perception that continues today. This perception is that they are members of a separate and troublesome social category — people who are distinct from and problematic to the living. It is in exclusion and the construction of boundaries that this association is most clearly seen. Boundaries have been a keen concern in the development of learning-disability services (Todd, Evans and Beyer, 1990) and although the exclusion of people with learning disabilities is important, there is:

> *an exclusion that precedes every other, more radical than the exclusion of madmen, children or inferior races, an exclusion preceding all these and serving as their model: the exclusion of the dead and of death... There is an irreversible evolution from savage societies to our own: little by little, the dead cease to exist. They are thrown out of... symbolic circulation.*
> Baudrillard (1993: 126)

People with learning disabilities, the dying and the dead, therefore, belong to worlds preoccupied with social and symbolic order. Furthermore, and perhaps more problematically, the learning disability world has used 'death' as a metaphor to make sense of and critique its history of approaches to learning disability. This critique suggests that the social response to learning disability has been to render people 'as-if' dead. This has been reversed so that it is life that is now valued and, in the process, the learning-disability community seems keen to 'escape' death.

Our attitudes and responses to death are far from constant. Aries (1976) has presented a history of distinctive death periods from mediaeval times to the late twentieth century. His analysis is that 'death' is not a static phenomenon, and that there are five epochs:

- tame death
- death of self
- remote or imminent death
- death of other
- invisible death.

There is little scope here to explore these five epochs in depth. For the purposes of this chapter, I will focus on the two chronological extremes, 'tame death' and 'invisible death'. These extremes are separated by the emergence of modern medicine and science, and the displacement of 'community' by 'privacy'. During this period, the concept of death as a familiar event becomes replaced by one that suppresses it. Death was commonplace, and therefore more visible and intimate, during the Middle Ages than it is today. From public executions to mass epidemics, from death-bed rituals to cemetery-based cultural exchanges, death was difficult to avoid or deny. In more recent times, there have been further changes in our attitudes to death and dying — changes that seek to reverse the distancing of dead and dying people.

Familiarity with death

In earlier times, death had a definite presence within life and was always within touching distance. Cemeteries, for example, were not then places of social exclusion or erasure: they were places of social, economic and cultural exchange. Aries describes how, in the seventeenth century, cemeteries were places for gamblers, jugglers, theatrical troops and musicians, and how these gatherings would take place alongside funeral services. Ghosts, according to the belief-system of the time, had the capacity to be both malevolent or munificent; it was also believed that the dead could pass into the world of the living. The recently dead were in a state that was between life and death. The point at which the spirit left the body was thought to be located some time after biological death, and many funerary customs were based on this belief (for example, helping the deceased make the transition safely to 'the other side'). Richardson (1987) examines the controversy caused by the 1832 Anatomy Act, which was to provide the corpses of paupers and the poor, the unclaimed dead of the poorhouse, for dissection. There was resistance to the Act owing to the popular belief that the connection between the soul and the body continued for an undefined period after death. Waking was also an important ritual that occurred on the eve of the funeral to ensure that death had taken place, as well as to ward off evil spirits that might mislead the soul when it eventually departed the body. Food or drink was often taken in the presence of the corpse as a means of removing sins from the deceased. Thus, many of the rituals associated with death were prefigured on the needs of the dead, not the living.

Memorial effigies of the dead also reminded the viewer of the nearness of death; and, in particular, of their own death. The 'transi', memorials depicting a decaying and decomposing body, were a form of 'memento mori' by which the living were reminded of the inevitability of death, and that death was not only present within life, but that it could occur at any hour (Kearle, 1989). Death had a visible presence and was something for which people were expected to be prepared. The recognition of individual mortality was well-illustrated in the *Artes Moriendi (The Art of Dying)*, an instructional manual that commanded: 'Therefore prepare without delay, For no-one knows his dying day'.

Exclusionary impulses

Yet this familiarity was about to cease and old ways of dealing with death were soon to be disrupted. Aries (1976) argues that our response to death and dying underwent a brutal historical revolution so that the dead and death would become annihilated and effaced. The dead and dying were increasingly 'pushed further behind the scenes [and]... isolated.' Slowly, and from the mid-nineteenth century to more recent times, the dead and dying were at worst displaced and at best made to be as unobtrusive as possible. Roach (1996) writes that the dead were compelled to leave the spaces of the living. This exclusion began with the 'necropolitan revolution' (Queiroz and Rugg, 2003) or the removal of places of disposal and burial to the outskirts of towns when previously local churchyards had sufficed. Although this move met with some resistance (Aries, 1976), the shift from churchyard to cemetery was done in the name of hygiene and public health, and was further facilitated by epidemics of cholera in the nineteenth century. The dead were contagious and burial grounds were considered to be places of evil (Murray, 2003). As Murray (2003: 135) quotes from a report of an Australian health officer in 1862:

It is a well established fact, that exhalations from the dead... may continue for many years... there are constant noxious emanations. The gases so evolved are of a most poisonous nature — and... have been known to destroy life — when the gases are more diluted with atmospheric air, they produced epidemic putrid disease.

There were changes in the style and function of remembrance that came to value and idealise 'life over death'. The 'transi' became a hideous form that signified a repulsion towards death or a form of life that lured the living to their untimely destruction. Decay was no longer to be the significant symbolic feature of the corpse and photography became a common way of capturing the images of the dead. Decay became repulsive. In these Victorian images, the recently dead were posed in their daily clothes as 'living' or 'asleep'. The living body was idealised even in death, thereby rendering death invisible and out of place. The corpse also came to be seen as having no connection with the soul, and funeral rites began to serve the needs of the bereaved rather than the deceased. The style of mourning changed because the objective was to return to normality as soon as possible: the dead, according to these new beliefs, should not leave a space and should not disrupt the business of life. As Walter (1997) argues, extended periods of mourning were only ever available for the upper and middle classes as the exigencies of surviving through waged-labour were more pressing for the working classes. However, for all social classes, the spaces left by the dead were to be filled by the needs of the living. A further divorce between the living and the dead was struck by the emergence of Protestantism, with its prohibition of indulgences and intermediaries (Walter, 1997). The growth of professional undertakers also added another boundary between the living and dead.

According to Blauner (1966), modern culture sought to put a clean break between the living and the dead, and thereby expurge death from life. As death could be further pushed to the later years, it became easier to remove death to a safe and distant zone. Over time, the point at which the dead are separated from the living has moved. In earlier times, the period shortly after death was the transitional period. Then, life vacated the body some days after death, before moving onto a new dimension of existence. Now, there exists the potential for the pre-mortem disintegration of identity and social removal. Whereas dying would typically have taken place at home, by the middle of the twentieth century dying was more likely to occur in hospital, a setting where death becomes an embarrassing medical and scientific failure that was best hidden. Indeed, as Glaser and Strauss (1967) point out, the status of dying was often hidden from the dying themselves. They are separated from the world of the living as a preparation for 'being dead'. Sociological studies described the impoverished experiences of dying and, in particular, their depersonalisation and segregation. Levine and Scotch (1970), for example, argue that the dying are treated as offensive and insulting. Sudnow (1967) describes the 'social death' of dying patients and how staff, as well as relatives, come to treat the dying as if they are already dead. Biological and social deaths are far from identical and the latter acknowledges that the social existence of an individual may be diminished or removed before they are biologically dead (Sudnow, 1967). Once, social death was thought to postdate biological death; in the twentieth century, however, social death occurs before biological death. As Aries (1976: 86–7) writes, this is done for the sensibilities of the living:

> *The dying person [is] rapidly covered over by a different sentiment, a news sentiment characteristic of modernity: one must avoid — no longer for the sake of the dying person, but for society's sake, for the sake of those close to the dying person — the disturbance and overly strong and unbearable emotion caused by the ugliness of dying and by the very presence of death in the midst of a happy life.*

More recently, Lawton (2000) has written of the nature of decline before death and how the deteriorating body and sense of self are linked before death. The civilised body is not only living, but also controlled and disciplined, and hygienically bounded from others. Thus, dying can also be repulsive. The dead and the dying became banished for their capacity to repulse and disrupt the living.

In the wake of the dead

The way society has responded to death offers an historical parallel to way it has responded to people with learning disabilities. The origins of the 'asylum era' lie in the nineteenth century (Scull, 1979). Although forms of provision had existed before this, the systematic provision of institutional care did not really begin until after the provision of poorhouses established by the 1832 Poor Laws, which came in to force the same year as the Anatomy Laws. Both the poorhouse and the asylum replaced traditional systems of local and family care within which disabled people were present in local communities. Gleeson (1997) argues that disabled people typically figured in the artistic representation of town and village life up to the eighteenth century. Disabled and non-disabled people lived side by side up to this point in time (Scull, 1979).

However, their growing geographical separation began with the growth of industrialisation and social upheavals and imperatives of capitalism. The rise of the institution coincided with the rise of urban cemeteries, and for both populations, public health was the major concern. There are many examples of the perception that the disabled were an abject population. For example, in 1912, the Massachusetts Medical Society commented that such people were 'a menace and a danger to the community' and 'carriers of venereal disease' (Sarason and Doris, 1969). They were seen as socially threatening, as morally destructive, and as posing a eugenic (genetic) threat. The physical bodies of people with learning disabilities were also depicted as abject in that they were poorly bounded because of incontinence or drooling. They were, in Tregold's (1908) view, 'hideous, repulsive creatures… and in their life and death are revealed the culminating and final manifestations of the neuropathic diathesis'. The disgust evoked by the disabled body seems as strong as the danger evoked by a decomposing corpse.

Within institutions, people with learning disabilities have been described as being made 'socially dead'. People with disabilities were unduly and eagerly removed from their communities to die symbolically within institutions, settings that could be characterised as the descendants of society's initial practices of social exclusion — cemeteries (Baudrillard, 1993). Certainly, that is how institutions came to be seen: as places of safe disposal. They have typically been characterised as 'dumping grounds' or 'bins'. There are anecdotes of families having masses of remembrance said for their relatives who were sent to or taken into institutional care.

Death has also provided a ready and shocking metaphor for sociologists and others who were critical of institutional models of care. Goffman (1961) wrote of the processes of 'mortification' whereby individuals were taken out of symbolic, as well as physical, circulation and disciplined to the imperatives of institutional life. This would cause the loss of a person's sense of self. The metaphor of death is also repeated in forceful fashion in Blatt and Kaplan's *A Christmas in Purgatory* (1966). Residential services for people with learning disabilities have been easily viewed as social cemeteries, places to which parents were once asked to send their offspring and to think of them as having died. Indeed, some mothers today remember how they were encouraged to do so. One mother, for example, recalled how a professional had told her: 'You know, if you want to move on and get on with your life, and leave Geraint here, we've got some sort of country place that children go to, and leave him here!' (Todd and Jones, 2003: 234). Parents have also been described as undergoing a form of 'bereavement' on the path to their successful adjustment (Bicknell, 1988).

The extent to which social death is separate from biological death is seen clearly in the ways in which people with learning disabilities have been socially treated, particularly during the period of institutionalisation. Sinason (1993) writes that people with learning disabilities 'breathe in a societal death wish'. Wolfensberger (1987) is more scathing in his identification of 'death' with 'people with learning disabilities'. For him, social practices towards disabled people are a form of 'deathmaking' at both physical and metaphysical levels. He defines deathmaking as:

> *Any actions or pattern of actions which either directly or indirectly bring about or hasten the death of a person or group. Deathmaking includes actions ranging all the way from explicit, overt and direct killing of another person to a very concealed and indirect killing that may take a long time to accomplish and be very difficult to trace.*
>
> Wolfensberger (1987: 1)

Wolfensberger cites a range of deathmaking practices towards people with learning disabilities, including social rejection, pharmacological or experimental abuse, material deprivation, abortion and genocide. It also includes surrounding devalued individuals with deathly images. He cites, as examples, the placement of services for people with learning disabilities close to sites associated with death, or the sending of condolence cards to parents on the birth of a disabled child. Thus, the dead, the dying and the learning-disabled have come to share a common fate of exclusion and banishment from the world of the living. Although the term 'social death' is a modern coinage used to describe how those close to dying are treated as if they were already dead, Mulchay (1993: 42) writes:

> *[it is] possible for extended social death sequences to stretch deeply back into people's existence as living organisms.*

Inclusive impulses

Society's way of dealing with the dead and with learning-disabled people continues to change, and these changes continue to show similarities. The dead and the dying are beginning to be re-located back into a new symbolic space, which parallels changes taking place in the relocation of people with learning disabilities. As ideas of an 'ordinary life' and 'inclusion' have become modern anthems for the learning-disability world, 'the good death' has provided much the same organising principles in modern approaches to death and dying within the palliative-care community. Both communities were founded on anti-institutional and anti-medical ethics. The institution became an inappropriate place for living or dying. Both movements were also founded on a radical critique of hospital care and the impersonal, medicalised and devaluing treatment individuals received (James, 1989; Twycross, 1986). The modern hospice movement developed, in the UK, in the late 1960s — just about the same time that institutions for people with learning disabilities were beginning their long demise. By 1995, in-patient hospice units and domiciliary provision for the dying had become well-established (Higginson, 1997). The same period witnessed the development of community-based residential, day and domiciliary programmes for people with learning disabilities (Felce *et al*, 1998). Lawton (2000: 12) writes how the hospice emphasises 'family, community affiliation and community responsibility' and promotes a particular view of self as active and participating. The modern hospice movement sought to bring to an end the pre-mortem disintegration of the self and to promote dying as a transitional period in which the individual ought to be seen as living and participating for as long as possible.

A core concern of the hospice movement has been the idea of a 'good death', an idea that enshrines humane relationships in personal control and choice. These views would be easily translated within the learning-disability community. The fundamental principles of an 'ordinary life' also stress equal human value and rights, individuality and participation within the community. Just as the dying were to be given some life for as long as possible, so too were people with learning disabilities being given similar pledges by their own reformers. However, whilst the hospice philosophy was based on an acceptance of death as a natural part of life, the learning-disability world seems to disavow death. Although both communities give value to life, in one (the learning-disability world) death is marginalised and continues to be hidden. The argument presented above suggests that death is treated this way because it has an uneasy and discomforting history within the world of learning disability. Death represents the darkest moments in the social history of learning disability, and perhaps it somehow haunts this community, reminding it of a time when death eclipsed life; it may thus be an association that is unwelcome and stigmatising. Furthermore, there is an obsession within learning-disability services over a range of aspects of living, for example, extended living, a good working life and the development of relationships. Death is almost a taboo — a shameful threat to the rationale for modern approaches to learning disability.

Yet although death may be denied as an inappropriate metaphor for learning disability, it cannot be escaped quite so easily. People with learning disabilities will one day be dead, and for many this may be preceded by a phase of dying. As Hockey (1988: 201) writes, in relation to homes for the elderly, 'death [is] always waiting in the wings'. Dying and the care of dying are enormously complex and challenging phenomena that we will not resolve by turning our backs on them. Yet, the reluctance of research and services to deal with this aspect of living may mean that many experience this phase in silent and unsupported apprehension. There is clearly a need for the learning-disability world to embrace death once again, at least in the way death impinges on individuals with learning disabilities, on relatives and on services.

Embracing death within life

Death is likely to be a challenging presence in the learning-disability world, but, as the brief historical review suggests, it may not be as unfamiliar as many people think. Furthermore, an engagement with it need not entail a denial of life. Although the relation between the worlds of the dead and people with a learning disability has been a long and disturbing one, this relation has made possible a more positive and direct form of collaboration — one based on shared principles and values. In this section of the chapter, I will outline areas for exploration.

Ordinary staffed houses are becoming the most common service setting for people with learning disabilities, and it is within such services that most people with learning disabilities enter the dying phase. However, such settings have not typically been associated with places of dying. Dying in such a setting is likely to be challenging for care staff, given that they are working in a 'life-orientated' service. How such settings attend to issues of dying and the demands this places on them are not at all understood. Studies of death in a variety of non-medical, non-palliative care services reveal a lack of staff training and preparation for death (Katz *et al*, 1999). Grande *et al* (1998) reveal that few elderly people with incurable chronic diseases are likely to be admitted into specialist palliative-care services. Evidence from research on residential services for older people in general suggests that non-palliative residential services are poorly prepared and resourced for dealing with dying residents, and that access to specialist palliative services can be also poor (Komarony, 2001; Zerzan *et al*, 2000). In two small-scale research studies based on opportunistic sampling, there is sufficient evidence that the dying phase in the lives of people with learning disabilities is problematic (Brown, Burns and Flynn, 2002; Todd, in press).

There is a clear need for palliative care involvement in helping learning disability services provide care for people who are dying. However, this service also has much to learn about providing services to people with learning disabilities who are dying and to their relatives and carers. Palliative care services are unfamiliar with the unique needs and challenges of specific groups (Oliviere and Monroe, 2004). There is a clear need for collaboration between these two spheres, one based on detailed and sound research of its impact.

Of course, death extends beyond professional spheres of influence to the dying individual and his or her family. Researchers may have typically found it hard to obtain the views of people with learning disabilities about their lives, but it will be even more challenging to discuss death with them. Services, too, may find this difficult (Todd, in press). Bereavement is one of the few aspects of death that has a presence within the learning-disability research field. This comes from correcting a longstanding inability to credit people with learning disabilities with shared humanity, and therefore with an emotional life. Oswin (1991) argues that despite the changes in attitudes and practices towards people with learning disabilities, there is still a significant problem in recognising that people with learning disabilities have an emotional self, which means that they do not receive support in the areas of loss and bereavement. Exclusion from participation in cultural rituals associated with death may place the individual at risk from more intense and problematic emotional angst. Learning-disabled people have been described as the forgotten people of the emotional world. As Read (1997: 5) writes:

For many years, people with a learning disability have had forgotten deaths, forgotten grief and have often become forgotten people when it comes to meaningful support over the death of a loved one.

If the learning-disability world finds it challenging to recognise death in the lives of people with learning disabilities, facing an individual with learning disabilities with news that they themselves are dying will also be fraught and difficult. Indeed, Todd (in press) reveals that few adults with learning disabilities who were dying were aware of what was happening to them. Without such knowledge, people cannot possibly be involved in decision-making towards the end of their lives.

It has been easy to overlook the fact that people living in service settings may remain embedded in a family network, even if they are not living at home. When an individual is dying, the role and presence of family members can be highly problematic for staff, and is an area for future research (Todd, in press). Furthermore, parents of children with learning disabilities are more likely than other parents to have to deal with the premature death of their children. The impact of a child's death on family relationships can be enormous, so the family's support needs can be enormous too (Riches and Lawson, 2000). However, these needs are poorly understood; indeed, some even argue that these families are 'disenfranchised' of their grief. There is evidence that the grief these parents experience is both overwhelming and unrecognised by others (Todd, in press).

What is needed is research that allows an examination of people's ancestry and continuing bonds after death (Walter, 2001). Research that adopts a 'death-as-part-of-life' perspective must also look beyond the pre-mortem period to the meaning of the deaths of learning-disabled people for those who survive them, and how their lives are remembered and commemorated.

Summary — letting death into life

Nobody should doubt the significance of death and dying for the learning-disability community. The issues of end-of-life care for these people are likely to be challenging and take the learning disability world by surprise. In this chapter, I have argued that there has been a close and sometimes explicit link between the worlds of learning disability and the dead — a link that the modern learning-disability community has sought to break in the name of progress and life. However, in so doing, I have argued, the lives of people with learning disabilities are devalued rather than affirmed. Yet the shared philosophical ground between the learning-disability and palliative-care communities must be cause for optimism in the future.

Dying is an unrecognised and difficult transition within the learning-disability world. If, as May (2001: 8) argues, the increasing use of the term 'transition' in learning-disability literature points to 'parallels between our lives and the lives of people with intellectual disabilities... [and their] shared concerns and experiences', the inclusion of dying or death makes the overlap more complete. Dying is the final realisation of this common ground, not its denial. To deny the relevance of death is to maintain, deliberately or otherwise, a practice of exclusion. If we belief that the lives of people with learning disabilities have the same value as other people's, so too must their deaths. More study and understanding of death is a necessary step for the learning-disability world, not only as a response to the needs of individuals who are dying and those who will grieve for them, but also as an important recognition that people with learning disabilities are a part of us, rather than being apart *from* us. Acceptance that people with learning disabilities will die and be remembered may be not the stamp of exclusion, be the final act of an ordinary life. Embracing death within our community is an act of inclusion which shows the value we attach to the lives and contributions of people with learning disabilities.

References

Aries P (1976) *Western Attitudes Towards Death*. Marion Boyars, London

Baudrillard J (1993) *Symbolic Exchange & Death*. Sage, London

Bicknell J (1988) The psychopathology of handicap. In: May D (ed) *Living with Mental Handicap: Transitions in the Lives of People with Mental Handicap*. Jessica Kingsley, London

Blatt B, Kaplan F (1966) *Christmas in Purgatory: a Photographic Essay in Mental Retardation*. Newton, Allyn & Bacon

Blauner R (1966) Death and social structure. *Psychiatry* **29**: 378–94

Brown H, Burns S, Flynn M (2002) Supporting people through terminal illness and death. In: *Today and Tommorrow*. Foundation for People with Learning Disabilties, London

Carter G, Jancar J (1983) Mortality in the mentally handicapped. *Am J Ment Defic* **27**: 143–56

Collman R, Stoller A (1963) Data on mongolism in Australia. *J Ment Defic Res* **7**: 60–8

Felce D, Grant G, Todd S, Ramcharan P, Beyer S, McGrath M, Perry P, Shearn J, Kilsby M, Lowe K (1998) *Towards a Full Life*. Butterworth-Heinemann, Oxford

Field D, Hockey J, Small N (1997) Making sense of difference: death, gender and ethnicity in modern Britain. In: Field D, Hockey J, Small N (eds) *Death, Gender & Ethnicity*. Routledge, London

Fryers T (1986) Survival in Down's Syndrome. *J Ment Defic Res* **30**: 101–10

Glaser BG, Strauss AL (1967) Awareness contexts and social interaction. *Am Sociol Rev* **29**: 669–79

Gleeson B (1999) *Geographies of Disability*. Routledge, London

Goffman E (1961) *Asylums*. Penguin, Harmondsworth

Grande GE, Addington-Hall JM, Todd CJ (1998) Place of death and access to home care services: are certain patient groups at a disadvantage? *Soc Sci Med* **47**: 565–79

Higginson I (1997) *Health Care Needs Assessment: Palliative and Terminal Care*. Radcliffe, Oxford

Hockey J (1988) Residential care and the maintenance of social identity. In: Jeffryes M (ed) *Growing Old in the Twentieth Century*. Routledge, London

James N (1994) Emotional labour. *Sociol Rev* **37**: 15–42

Jancar J, Eastham R, Carter G (1984) Hypnocholeseterolaemia in cancer and other causes of death in the mentally handicapped. *Br J Psychiatry* **145**: 59–61

Katz J, Komarony C, Siddell M (1999) Understanding palliative care in residential and nursing homes. *Int J Palliat Nurs* **5**: 58–64

Kearle M (1989) *Endings: a Sociology of Death and Dying*. OUP, New York

Komorony C (2002) The performance of the hour of death. In: Hockley J, Clark D (eds) *Palliative Care for Older People in Care Homes*. Open University Press, Buckingham

Lawton J (2000) *The Dying Process*. Routledge, London

Levine S, Scotch N (1970) Dying as an emerging social problem. In: Brim OG (ed) *The Dying Patient*. Russel Sage, New York

Lovell A (1997) Death at the beginning of life. In: Field D, Hockey J, Small N (eds) *Death, Gender & Ethnicity*. Routledge, London

May D (2001) *Living with Mental Handicap: Transitions in the Lives of People with Mental Handicap*. Jessica Kingsley, London

McEnhill L (2004) Disability. In: Oliviere D, Monroe B (eds) *Death, Dying and Social Differences*. Oxford University Press, Oxford

Mulkay M (1993) Social death in Britain. In: Clark D (ed) *The Sociology of Death*. Blackwell, Oxford

Murray L (2003) Modern innovations? Ideal vs reality in colonial cemeteries of 19th century New South Wales. *Mortality* **8**: 129–43

Oliviere D, Monroe B (eds) Introduction: working with death, dying and difference. In: Oliviere D, Monroe B (eds) *Death, Dying and Social Differences*. Oxford University Press, Oxford

Oswin M (1991) *Am I Allowed to Cry?* Souvenir Press, London

Patja K (2001) *Life Expectancy and Mortality in Intellectual Disability*. FAMR Publications, Helsinki

Queiroz F, Rugg J (2003) The development of cemeteries in Portugal. *Mortality* **8**: 113–38

Read S (1997) A sense of loss: working with loss and people who have a learning disability. *Nurs Stand Learning Unit* (Suppl) 071 11: 36

Riches G, Lawson P (2000) *An Intimate Loneliness*. Open University Press, Buckingham

Richardson R (1987) *Death, Dissection and the Destitute*. Routledge and Kegan Paul, London

Roach J (1996) *Cities of the Dead*. Columbia University Press, New York

Sarason SB, Doris J (1979) *Educational Handicap, Public Policy and Social History*. Macmillan, New York

Scull A (1979) *Museums of Madness: the Social Organisation of Insanity in Nineteenth-century England*. St Martin's Press, New York

Similia S (1986) Mortality of mentally retarded children to 17 years of age assessed in a prospective one-year birth cohort. *J Ment Defic Res* **30**: 401–5

Sinason V (1993) *Mental Handicap and the Human Condition*. Free Association, London

Sudnow D (1967) *Passing On: the Social Organization of Dying*. Prentice Hall, Englewood Cliffs, NJ

Todd S (in press) *Memento Mori: So People with Learning Disabilities Die?* Welsh Centre for

Learning Disabilities, Cardiff, Wales

Todd S (2002) Death does not become us. *J Gerontol Soc Work* **38**: 225–40

Todd S, Evans G, Beyer S (1990) More recognised than known. *Aust New Zealand J Develop Disabil* **16**: 207–18

Todd S, Jones S (2003) Mum's the word. *J Appl Res Intellect Disabil* **16**: 229–244

Tregold A (1908) *Mental Defiency: Amentia.* Balliere, Tindal and Cox, London

Twycross R (1986) *A Time to Die.* Christian Medical Fellowship, London

Walter T (1991) Modern death: taboo or not taboo? *Sociology* **25**: 293–310

Walter T (1997) *On Bereavement: the Culture of Grief.* Open University Press, Buckingham

Wolfensberger (1987) *The New Genocide of Handicapped and Afflicted People.* Syracuse University Division of Special Education and Rehabilitation, Syracuse, USA

Zerzan J, Stearns S, Hanson L (2000) Access to palliative care and hospices in nursing homes. *JAMA* **284**: 2489–94

CHAPTER 3

How did you cope? Learning from case studies in death and dying

Jacqueline Furniss, Heather Morris, Sue Read

The diagnosis of a palliative illness for anyone is one of the most traumatic life experiences, both for the person who has been diagnosed and for friends and family around them. For a person with a learning disability to receive a diagnosis of a palliative illness (or for one of their loved ones to receive such a diagnosis) is equally distressing. The World Health Organisation (WHO) (1990: 11) defines palliative care as 'the active total care of patients whose disease is not responsive to curative treatment. Control of pain, of other symptoms and of psychological, social and spiritual problems is deemed paramount. The goal of palliative care is the achievement of the best quality of life for patients and their families'. This definition puts great emphasis on quality of life until death.

The UK Department of Health (DoH) (2001) defines learning disability as including the presence of impaired intelligence with impaired social functioning that began before adulthood and which has a lasting effect on development. Tuffrey-Wijne (2003) suggest that because of the increased longevity of individuals with learning disabilities, they are more likely to require palliative care services in the future. Those who are given a dual diagnosis of palliative care and learning disabilities may present with a range of challenges, which are often present at various levels throughout their enduring illness. Additionally, other practical, social, ethical, spiritual and moral considerations may be involved as a variety of professionals seek to offer appropriate palliative care and support to this minority population.

Disempowerment is a common issue for all people experiencing a palliative illness, but specifically for people with learning disabilities, who are often excluded from being involved in death and dying and are often not informed of the death (or impending death) of their loved ones (Oswin, 2001). People with a learning disability may also have communication difficulties (Kerr *et al*, 1996), which may result in the delay of the initial diagnosis, as symptoms are often masked and go unnoticed. This delay in diagnosis may often result in a poor prognosis (Tuffrey – Wijne, 1997). Generic care services may find that when trying to provide pain and symptom control for this group of people, communication problems will present a significant barrier to treatment. Subsequently, people with learning disabilities are often perceived as being vulnerable regarding death and dying (Read and Elliot, 2003).

All the factors above will affect the way people with learning disabilities are supported through any palliative illness. The two case studies presented in this chapter draw on the personal and professional experiences of the authors. They will provide insight into a range of dilemmas and challenges that could be faced, either by the individual with a learning disability who is experiencing a palliative illness, or by the same person being confronted with the pending death of a parent and sole, primary carer. Issues surrounding the professional care and support will also be explored.

People with learning disabilities endure palliative illness in the same way as the general population (Read, 1998a) and this is reflected in the increase in available literature on this specialist subject (Keenan and McIntosh, 2000; Tuffrey-Wijne, 1997; Lindop and Read, 2000). There is a wealth of literature on general palliative care (eg. Copp, 1999; Parkes *et al*, 1996) and case studies are often a popular method within such research.

Qualitative research methods are suitable for studying many aspects of palliative nursing practice generally, and specifically with regard to people with learning disabilities (Bycroft, 1994). Burns and Grove (1997) define qualitative research as a systematic, subjective approach to describing life experiences and giving them meaning. Platt (1998) describes case studies as being contextual and holistic, and since palliative care is defined as involving a holistic approach (WHO, 1990), case studies are an appropriate methodological choice. Case studies often add a richness to the research dialogue, are easy to relate to, are informative, and are a way of meaningfully linking theoretical perspectives to clinical practice.

For the purpose of this chapter, the authors will use two case studies to explore specific situations and experiences of palliative care involving people with learning disabilities. Case studies focus on the lived experiences of individuals and give a flavour of the issues faced by those involved; they are, therefore, ideally suited as a tool to explore palliative care issues generally and specifically in the arena of people with learning disabilities. The two case studies offered are not deemed to be representative of all palliative care issues with this client population, but are used to illustrate the diversity of issues that may be faced by individuals and their carers. The case studies will also indicate the importance of effective communication. As Lee states, 'a prerequisite for good care is good communication' (1995: 54).

Aims

The overall aim of this chapter, then, is to explore the issues involved when the person with a learning disability experiences a palliative illness, either directly or indirectly. Specifically, the chapter aims to:

1. Compare and contrast two case studies to identify common and differing issues.
2. Consider the needs of people with a learning disability from within a general palliative care perspective.
3. Promote positive practice through shared dialogues and experiences.

The case studies

All names and circumstances have been changed in the case studies to protect confidentiality. The first case study provides an example of the complexities of care issues involved in bereavement and anticipatory death for a man with learning disabilities. The second case study illustrates the issues involved when an individual with a learning disability receives a personal diagnosis of a palliative condition.

Analysis of the case studies

Despite their differences, the two case studies (*3.1*: Bob and *3.2*: Leanne) share certain similarities, which are consistent with palliative care in general. The authors independently analysed both case studies, compared their findings, and identified six emergent core themes (*Table 3.1*).

Case Study 3.1: Bob

Bob is a forty-two year-old man who has a learning disability and manageable challenging behaviours. Bob lived at home with his seventy-six year-old father, Jim. His mother had died thirteen years previously in a local hospice after a long illness. Before his mother's death, Bob had attended a local Day Service but, following the family bereavement, chose to stay at home. Although Jim had been a fit and healthy man, one of the reasons that Bob gave for staying at home was 'just in case my father feels poorly'. Jim had recently been feeling unwell and his GP had sent him for a series of tests at the local hospital.

Bob had an older sister, Elsie, who lived nearby with her husband. Elsie was becoming increasingly concerned about Bob's isolation and what would happen in the future because, as she put it, 'none of us are spring chickens'. Following a family discussion, Elsie contacted the Adult Social Worker Duty Officer, who made an initial visit to the family prior to the case being allocated to a social worker. The Duty Officer also referred the case to the MENCAP Sharing Caring Project Coordinator, who is also a Registered Nurse for People with Learning Disabilities. This project offered support and information to older carers in the local area.

The Project Coordinator visited the family three days after the referral. Bob stayed in his bedroom during this time, as he felt uncertain of strangers. Jim repeatedly told the coordinator that the family were 'fine' and did not need any help. Elsie raised her concerns for the future and also explained that she was worried that Bob still talked to his mother. Jim explained that at the time he had felt it best to tell Bob that his mother 'was on holiday' and he had never been told he truth about her death. Bob still talks about his mother and often says that he wishes she would come home. Although, while talking to the family, the MENCAP worker had been concerned about some aspects of the case, she had not felt that the first visit was an appropriate time to begin to address the issues and that she first needed to work at developing a trusting relationship with the family, particularly Jim.

The day before the coordinator was due to make her second visit to the family, she received a phone call from Elsie who told her that Jim had visited his GP earlier that week, and the GP had broken the news to Jim that he had cancer of the liver and that there was no active treatment. Elsie was obviously very upset, but she said that the family had decided that as far as possible Jim would be cared for at home and that Bob would remain in the family home at least until Jim had 'passed away'. Jim had asked Elsie to ask the Project Coordinator to discuss ways of supporting Bob through his father's illness when she visited the family on the following day.

Case Study 3.2: Leanne

Leanne was a seventy-four year-old woman with a learning disability who had lived in residential care for seven years. Before this she had spent forty years in a long-stay institution, and had been resettled in 1993, together with two long-standing friends.

Leanne was diagnosed with secondary carcinoma of the lungs after six months of investigations. The main reason for the delay in diagnosis was Leanne's reluctance to display or communicate any pain. The initial carcinoma had been diagnosed seven years previously, which resulted in the removal of a kidney. Hospital treatment was a long-standing cause of anxiety to Leanne, as she had a phobia of illness, death and hospitals, which was believed to originate in previous experiences when her mother had died. The majority of care was provided in her home environment by the care team, which was composed of one Registered Nurse and seven care staff. Although the care staff had considerable experience in learning disabilities, they had limited knowledge of palliative care issues,.

It was decided from the onset of the diagnosis and prognosis of Leanne's condition that she would continue to be cared for in her home environment by familiar care staff. This was achieved by using the knowledge of a wide range of health professional and palliative care experts. The sense of intrusion into Leanne's life was minimised by the care manager liaising between the professionals and Leanne, thereby facilitating the palliative care offered.

On several occasions, an ethics forum discussed difficult issues relating to Leanne's anxieties over hospitals. Leanne also had a history of being a so-called 'faddy eater', so as her illness progressed, those on the forum were involved in the debate as to whether her lack of appetite was in fact a product of existing behaviours or her illness.

Leanne lived with her illness for eighteen months, as did the care team. Throughout the progression of her illness, the main focus for the care team was to ensure that Leanne's dignity was maintained at all times.

Discussion

Truth-telling in a palliative care context is a recurring issue (McLoughlin, 1989). Breaking bad news to any individual is often difficult, but when that individual has a learning disability, these problems are often multiple and complex (Read, 1998b). As a result, withholding information about death and dying is common among the carers of people with learning disabilities (McLaughlin, 1989).

Bob (*Case Study 1*) had never been told that his mother had died; he was told only that she had 'gone on holiday'. Oswin (2001) highlighted the fact that, historically, people with learning disabilities had often been shielded from death and denied the opportunity to grieve because they have not been told the truth. Naturally, Bob continued to talk about and miss his mother. Bob had lost his mother, although he had not been told of any of the circumstances around her disappearance from his life. Complicated grief reactions are often caused by factors and circumstances surrounding the death (Fisher and Warman, 1996) and the loss of his mother may have caused Bob to grieve. However, this grief has still not been resolved. People with learning

Table 3.1: Themes across case studies 3.1 (Bob) and 3.2 (Leanne)

Sex, age in years	Circumstance	Context of care	Care coordination	Professionals involved	Communication issues	Truth-telling
Bob						
Male, 42	Impending death of main carer.	Lived at home with his father.	The family currently coordinate the care for Bob and his father.	Currently only the project coordinator (RNMH). Father's palliative illness will mean that a variety of professionals will become involved.	History of poor communication from the family. Overprotection. Communication challenge between Bob and the project coordinator.	Bob has not been told the truth about his mother's death. Dealing with his father's impending death. Breaking bad news (who? when? how?)
Leanne						
Female, 74	Impending death due to cancer.	Lived in residential home for people with learning disabilities. Spent a brief time in respite at a local hospice.	Care cocoordinated by the care manager (RNME), liaising with all experts and providing Leanne with information.	Care manager. Support workers. District Nurse. GP/Consultant/ Marie Curies Nurses. Douglas Macmillan Nurses. Funeral Director. Ethics committee. Dietician.	Leanne was reluctant to express her feelings/pain. Leanne needed information, explaining to her in a way she could understand. Communication with the other people in the house. Communication with the care team.	Difficult because of existing phobias. Issues relating to diagnosis.

disabilities are often disenfranchised grievers (Doka, 1989) in as much that they are not allowed to grieve openly for there loved ones.

Telling Leanne (*Case Study 2*) of her diagnosis raised concerns because she had a long-standing phobia of illness, death and hospitals that had stemmed from the death of her mother several years before. The care team were very aware that, whilst they did not want to withhold any vital information from Leanne, they also did not want to overload her with information she did not want or that would be detrimental to her psychological and emotional well-being. Advice was sought from a bereavement counsellor, familiar with the client group, and the issues were subsequently discussed at a multidisciplinary ethics forum. A decision was made that familiar care staff would provide Leanne with as much information as she requested. Allowing the pace to be determined by Leanne meant that only the information she wanted would be offered. It was agreed that certain words that were known to cause her distress were not to be used at all unless instigated by her (eg. 'death' would be replaced by a phrase such as 'we cannot cure your illness'). This was a multidisciplinary and balanced decision based on the emotional and psychological needs of the person who was dying. Above all, it was decided that nothing would be withheld from Leanne if she asked. Interestingly, throughout her illness, Leanne asked various question concerning her health, but never asked if she was dying.

Providing information to Leanne's friends in the home was also important. Whilst the care team was aware that her friends all needed honest and accurate information, they did not want to share knowledge that was not known to Leanne herself through personal choice. Again, the bereavement counsellor was involved in talking to, and working with, her friends. The majority of the preparation with her friends took place when Leanne's illness progressed so that there was physical evidence of her deteriorating condition (ie. confinement to bed). At this time, questions were asked and issues could be dealt with both individually and as a group.

A specialist bereavement counsellor may be required to explore sensitive issues with Bob (Elliot, 1995). His father was dying and this will probably be a painful and emotional time for him. The previous unresolved grief following the loss of his mother may subsequently have an effect on how he deals with his current experience.

The role of the bereavement counsellor was developed during Leanne's illness (*Case Study 2*), not only to support the care staff's decision-making processes, but also gradually to become involved in the day-to-day life of Leanne and her friends within the home. A gradual introduction of any new person was essential to ensure Leanne's acceptance. Read *et al* (1999) explain how a bereavement counsellor's role encompasses not only support and counselling from a bereavement perspective, but also a role in helping associated carers cope with palliative and terminal illnesses. In this case, the bereavement counsellor formed a friendship with Leanne by regularly calling in for 'a coffee and a chat', rather than any formal structured counselling sessions. This enabled Leanne to discuss issues in a safe and unthreatening manner and at a pace determined by herself. During these times, Leanne discussed issues that were important to her (not necessarily relating to her illness) that enabled the care team to plan for her future and, ultimately, her funeral.

A bereavement counsellor also facilitated regular sessions with the care team, where everyone was encouraged to express their anxieties, concerns and fears over any aspect of the care they were jointly undertaking. These informal sessions were held away from the home environment.

Other key professional issues included managing the tension between carers, family, friends and individual client needs, and maintaining open channels of communication with all parties to ensure everyone's interests were upheld. During his father's illness, Bob's family members hoped that they would both stay at the family home. As his father's condition worsened, this increased the need for more professional care input for father. This meant a number of health professionals visiting the home on a regular basis. Bob was uncertain of strangers and required a lot of support during this time. Bob may have decided not to stay at home during his father's illness, and it was important that Bob's needs and wishes were also considered. However, Bob's family's needs and wishes, particularly those of his father, must also be addressed. It should be remembered that the other family members were going through a very emotional and stressful time. Bob's father was going to lose his life and Elsie was going to lose her father. They will have their own grief to cope with, and may need emotional as well as practical support. At times, managing this tension may be very difficult, as everyone's needs and wishes will not always be the same, at the same time.

For people with learning disabilities who have communication difficulties too, it is essential to explore other methods of communication to facilitate choice and to ensure an individual's dignity is upheld. Good communication between personal carers and all professionals involved is needed to ensure that the best treatment, and appropriate support, is provided, especially in the sensitive area of death and dying.

One problem faced by the care team in *Case Study 2* was Leanne's reluctance to express or show that she was in pain, which meant that obtaining an accurate assessment was always difficult. Biersdorff (1994) reports that people with learning disabilities sometimes display hyperactive behaviour (rather than pain behaviour) to indicate medical needs. Such a change in behaviour was apparent with Leanne. She had always been a very 'particular' woman with respect to her personal hygiene and appearance. Suddenly, these behavioural patterns changed: she became reluctant to bath and lost interest in having her hair set, which she had previously insisted was done regularly. Although these changes were significant to the care team, they did not amount to evidence that could be acted on by other healthcare professionals. It was only when other physiological symptoms began to emerge several months later that tests could be undertaken and a diagnosis of carcinoma of the lining of the lung be reached. The focus then changed to helping Leanne to die a 'good death'. Hockey and Clarke (2002) have highlighted twelve principles of good practice to ensure a 'good death', which recognises that individual patients need to:

1. Know when death is coming and understand what can be expected.
2. Be able to retain control of what happens.
3. Be afforded dignity and privacy.
4. Have control over pain-relief and other symptom-control.
5. Have choice and control over where death occurs (at home or elsewhere).
6. Have access to information and expertise of whatever kind is required.
7. Have access to any spiritual or emotional support required.
8. Have access to hospice care in any location, not only in hospital.
9. Have control over who is present and who shares the end.
10. Be able to issue advance directives that ensure wishes are respected.
11. Have time to say goodbye and have control over other aspects of timing.
12. Be able to leave when it is time to go, and not have life prolonged pointlessly.

Dignity for Leanne was always a focal point for the care team. It is difficult enough to maintain any individual's dignity when physiological problems make intrusion necessary. Enes (2003) states that in the area of death and dying, dignity remains a poorly defined and unexplored concept, so that when the individual concerned has a learning disability, issues of control and independence become more complex challenges that incorporate communication barriers and cognitive abilities. It was at this time that the care manager played a pivotal role in liasing between all professionals involved in Leanne's care. As Pokorny's (1989) study showed, there is a definite link between a patient's dignity and the care and competence of the nurse. Enes (2003) defined dignity as 'being valued as a human being but related to having an individual significance and to be part of one's own unique world'. Minimising the intrusion into Leanne's life and maintaining routines and activities that she valued contributed to the maintenance of her dignity. By educating the care team within the home on various clinical procedures and methods of care, Leanne was able to maintain her privacy, only needing familiar staff to manage delicate and sensitive issues.

Forward planning may be an indicative part of palliative care for people with learning disabilities. Plans needed to be put into place for Bob's future care and this would generate several questions: where would Bob live after his father's death? If Bob decided to move, should this move be sooner rather than later? What does Bob ultimately want and what does the family want for Bob? Should Bob decide to move from the family home, he will endure further losses in addition to the loss of his father, including loss of routine, familiarity, neighbours and friends.

In Leanne's situation, the planning began at diagnosis, at the residential home for people with a learning disability, where she lived. Whilst the care team were experienced in caring for people with learning disabilities, they had little knowledge of palliative care. One of the first priorities for the care manager was to anticipate what services Leanne would need and identify where these could be accessed, should they be required in the future.

In consideration of the short- and long-term care-planning of Leanne, from the onset of her condition it was decided that she would be cared for in her home environment. Lee (1995) argues that being at home allows the individual a greater opportunity to determine his or her own care. When profound changes are taking place within the body and life, the consistency and familiarity of the home environment become particularly important. This was compounded in Leanne's case by the fact that she saw her current home as the only real home she had ever had as she had spent forty years sharing a ward in an institution. Her own personal bedroom and possessions and, more importantly, her pet cat were the most important things in her life.

Subsequently, the initial contact for assistance was made to the District Nurse through the General Practitioner. This individual became a vital and key link to initiating the contact between the care manager and the multidisciplinary team who eventually provided palliative care and support for Leanne. Corner (2003) states that although there is an agreement as to what constitutes palliative care, there is a less obvious consensus over what constitutes a palliative care team — although she does say that palliative care is best provided by the multidisciplinary team where the person and family remain the central focus. Opie (1997) believes that 'bringing together knowledge from different professionals and from clients in order to allow these differently sited knowledges to interrogate each other' may be the most fruitful way of facilitating a multidisciplinary team. In Leanne's case, she remained the central focus, but due to the communication difficulties and phobias concerned, the care manager's role became that of facilitating Leanne's access to all the information and advice received from a wide range of health professionals (*Table 3.1*) in a language and format that was simple, understandable and less intimidating.

In Bob's case, although the project coordinator was a Registered Nurse for people with learning disabilities, her role in her present position was to support the carer. Therefore, although Bob's needs and wishes were important when considering the support the carer needed, there was a requirement for other professionals to be involved to offer Bob the practical and emotional support he required. Referrals to a social worker, a community learning disability nurse and an independent advocate were required.

Part of the role of the MENCAP worker was to build a trusting relationship with the carers. In this case, Bob's father was experiencing a painful and emotional time and to build a relationship with him in this situation was a difficult but crucial task. As Jim's illness progressed, there would be other professionals involved in his care and it was important that Jim trusted the coordinator as plans were made and put into action for Bob's future.

Managing two issues — the father's impending death and Bob's future — meant the involvement of a multidisciplinary team, providing support for the father and support for Bob. When a large team of professionals are involved, the need for coordination of care is important. The question of who coordinates the care needs to be addressed, as this will promote both consistency and continuity of care. Jim's death will inevitably have an impact on the family, but by acting in a proactive manner and beginning to prepare the family, this impact can be reduced.

Conclusion and recommendations

This chapter has compared and contrasted two case studies and considered the needs of people with learning disability who require palliative care. The case studies promote positive practice in palliative care with this client group. The issues that have been highlighted and discussed are similar to the issues that arise in many palliative-care situations. However, there are complex and specific issues around each case as a direct result of the nature and context of learning disability.

Case studies, as a methodological approach, are useful vehicles from which to explore individual palliative-care experiences. Every palliative care situation is unique, as is each individual. The individuals within the two case studies are not presented as typical examples, since death and grief are unique and both occur in individual contexts. The complexity of the issues around these cases has generated a number of professional themes for the care teams involved. Issues related to communication, barriers to effective communication, truth-telling, the promotion of dignity and planning individualised care are present in both dialogues, and will also be important in general palliative care setting (Enes, 2003; Corner, 2003).

Hockey and Clarke's (2002) twelve principles that help ensure a 'good death' are directly transferable when providing palliative care for people with learning disabilities. The main difference will be *how* the information and options are communicated to the individuals concerned. The methods used to inform individuals may need to be adapted to ensure understanding, facilitate choice, and promote empowerment. By incorporating these principles into each individual's plan of care, an empathetic and holistic approach to palliative care can be achieved.

Accurate communication is crucial to all aspects of palliative care. From referral to diagnosis through to treatment options and prognosis — and, ultimately, death — communication will play an important role. Issues surrounding masked illness, resulting in delayed diagnosis; recognising the subtle behaviours that indicate distress; and promoting dignity and empowerment throughout the progression of the illness will all involve communication. Being familiar with the individual and having a knowledge of the associated issues relating to learning disability are paramount.

To assist in this, Tuffrey-Wijne (1997) suggests that close cooperation between the health professionals involved would ensure that maximum care and support are achieved.

Identifying one individual to coordinate or facilitate the care of the multidisciplinary palliative care team was found to be useful. This facilitator would coordinate care; would filter carers (to reduce the stress when the input of strangers would have caused undue anxiety to the individual concerned); and take responsibility for maintaining continuity of care. The situation was managed in both cases by the RNMH involved.

Ultimately, to reduce intrusion, a package of well-coordinated palliative care is essential. Within learning disability services 'learning disability nurses continue to have a pivotal role in coordination and delivering palliative care' (Read, 2003). Hunt and Wainwright (1994) recognised how the role of the nurse has changed over recent years and stated that there was a growing tendency for nurses to assume responsibility for many aspects of patient care, including palliative care. Subsequently, it would seem imperative to have nurses who have a duel qualification in both palliative care and learning disabilities.

References

Biersdorff K (1994) Incidence of significantly altered pain experience among individuals with developmental disabilities. *Am J Ment Retard* **98**: 619–31

Burns N, Groves S (1997) *The Practice of Nursing Research Conduct: Critique & Utilization.* WB Saunders Company, Pennsylvania

Bycroft L (1994) Care of a handicapped woman with metastic breast cancer. *Br J Nurs* **3**(3): 126–33

Copp G (1999) *Facing Impending Death: Experiences of Patients and their Nurses.* Nursing Times Books, London

Corner J (2003) The multidisciplinary team: fact or fiction? *Eur J Palliat Care* **10**(2): 10–13

Department of Health (DoH) (2001) *Valuing People: a New Strategy for Learning Disability for the 21ˢᵗ Century.* DoH, London

Doka KJ (ed) (1989) *Disenfranchised Grief L: Recognising Hidden Sorrow.* Lexington, Lexington MA

Elliot D (1995) Helping people with learning disabilities to handle grief. *Nurs Times* **91**(43): 27–9

Fisher M, Warman J (1990) *Bereavement and Loss: a Skills Companion.* The National Extension College, Cambridge

Hockney J, Clarke D (2002) *Facing Death: Palliative Care for Older People in Care Homes.* Open University Press, Berkshire

Hunt G, Wainwright P (1994) *Expanding the Role of the Nurse.* Blackwell Science, Oxford

Kerr M, Fraser W, Felce D (1996) Primary healthcare needs for people with a learning disability. *Br J Learn Disabil* **24**: 2–8

Keenan P, McIntosh P (2000) Learning disabilities and palliative care. *Palliat Care Today* P11–13

Lee E (1995) *A Good Death — Guide for Patients and Carers Facing Terminal Illness at Home.* Rosendale Press, London

Lindop E, Read S (2000) District Nurses' needs: palliative care for people with learning disabilities. *Int J Palliat Nurs* **6**(3): 117–122

McLoughlin J (1989) Bereavement in the mentally handicapped. *Br J Hosp Med* **36**(4): 256–60

Oswin M (2001) *Am I Allowed To Cry?* Human Horizons Series, Souvenier Press, London

Opie A (1997) Thinking teams and thinking clients: issues of disclosure and representation in the work of healthcare teams. *Sociol Health Illn* **19**(3): 259–80. Cited in: Corner J (2003) The multidisciplinary team: fact or fiction? *Eur J Palliat Care* **10**(2): 10–13

Parkes CM, Relf M, Couldrick A (1996) *Counselling in Terminal Care and Bereavement.* BPS Books, Leicester

Platt J (1998) What can case studies do? *Studies Qualit Methodol* **1**: 2–23. Cited in: Holloway I, Wheeler S (1996) *Qualitative Research for Nurses.* Blackwell Science, Oxford

Pokorny ME (1989) The Effects of Nursing Care on Human Dignity in the Critically Ill. PhD thesis, University of Virginia, USA, cited in: Enes S (2003) An exploration of dignity in palliative care. *Palliat Med* **17**: 263–9

PhD Thesis, University of Virginia. Cited in: Enes S (2003) An exploration of dignity in palliative care. *Palliat Med* **17**: 263–9

Read S (1996) How counselling services can help deal with loss and change. *Nurs Times* **92**: 38–40

Read S (1998a) The palliative care needs of people with learning disabilities. *Int J Palliat Nurs* **27**: 99–104

Read S (1998b) Breaking bad news to people with a learning disability. *Br J Nurs* **7**(2): 86–91

Read S, Frost I, Messenger N, Oates S (1999) Bereavement counselling and support for people with a learning disability: identifying issues and exploring possibilities. *Br J Learn Disabil* **27**(3): 99–104

Read S (2003) Bereavement and loss. Cited in: Markwick A, Parrish A (2003) *Learning Disabilities: Themes and Perspectives.* Butterworth Heinemann, Edinburgh

Read S, Elliot D (2003) Death and learning disability: a vulnerability perspective. *J Adult Protect* **5**(1): 5–14

Sumaya-Smith H (1995) Caregiver/resident relationships: surrogate family bonds and surrogate grieving in a skilled nursing facility. *J Adv Nurs* **21**: 447–51

Tuffrey-Wijne I (1997) Palliative care and learning disabilities. *Nurs Times* **93**(31): 50–1

Tuffrey-Wijne I (2003) The palliative care needs of people with intellectual disabilities: a literature review. *Palliat Med* **17**: 55–62

World Health Organisation (WHO) (1990) *Cancer Pain Relief and Palliative Care Report of WHO Expert Committee Series 804.* WHO, Geneva

CHAPTER 4

Pain and symptom management

Claud Regnard, Charlotte L Clarke, Lynn Gibson, Dorothy Matthews

In this chapter, we have outlined some of the key clinical issues to be considered in the symptom-management of people with learning disability who require palliative care. In so doing, we have sought to emphasise that the management of physical and psychological symptoms needs to take place within the context of a relationship between the individual and those caring for them. This is entirely consistent with the view of George and Sykes (1997) that palliative care's primary philosophy is the care of the whole person: 'It is not reductive, but divergent, exploring the roots and branches of a person's suffering, pain or distress. It is therefore labour-intensive, time-consuming and based in trusting relationships with patient and family'.

We have sought to rise to the challenge posed by Corner and Dunlop (1997) to allow the patient's narrative to surface. In this chapter, we have woven together the experience of one person, Ben, with the management of his symptoms. In so doing, we have had to dissect his experiences into a series of symptoms.

However, it has been necessary to imagine his thoughts, since Ben had very minimal communication ability, with no dis cernible speech and no sign language. His words have been written by his team to match his reactions to the problems he was experiencing.

Identifying distress

Ben's story

My name is Ben, I'm thirty-three years-old, and I've lived in this hospital for a very long time. I have a learning disability, some physical disabilities, and moving is difficult for me. I can't use words, but I can make my needs known by moving my eyes and hands. Today, my care manager has been to see me to tell me that a new home has been found for me and that I'll go to live there with some of my friends when everything gets sorted out. I'm really pleased, as I like being with people and am looking forward to living with my friends in a nice house instead of this big hospital ward.

I haven't been feeling well recently, and every time the nurses help me it's very uncomfortable for me, although they're always gentle. I heard the nurses say that my trousers are getting too big for me. I don't understand why, but the trouble is there are so many different staff working on my ward and a lot of them are new, so it's difficult for me to let them know how I feel about all the things that seem to be happening to me just now.

Distress is a complex state. A sense of being out of control and a lack of understanding of what is happening to oneself is both the cause and the consequence of distress. Someone who is distressed is often unable to pinpoint the reason for their distress, and this is compounded when the distress is experienced by someone with severe impairment of communication. While distress may have been caused by physical, psychological, spiritual or emotional issues in their lives, it is very likely to be expressed in a way that involves all of these domains. For example, a physical pain may result in a distress that causes fear, social withdrawal and increasingly poor self-esteem. This makes it more difficult for someone else to assess that person and identify their distress.

Ben's story points to two key factors. First, the many different staff make it hard for Ben to communicate with them all as an individual. If staff are to identify that Ben is in a distressed state, they need to know what he is like when he is not distressed — that is, they need a detailed knowledge of Ben himself. It is insufficient for them to have a knowledge only of working with people with a learning disability. Second, there needs to be continuity of care, so that services are organised in a way that makes it possible for staff to have a sustained relationship with Ben.

Identifying the causes of distress

Ben's story (continued)

Things aren't good today — I caused trouble at physiotherapy because I shouted loudly all of the time and tried to hit one of the staff. She became annoyed and took me back to the ward. But my back is sore and I didn't want to stand up in the special frame. And another thing — my cough isn't getting any better and my clothes are getting bigger! What's happening to me? One of the nurses is trying to get the GP to come back and examine me again, as one of my testicles is red, swollen and sore. I hope he comes today; he might know what to do. Doctors are clever people, aren't they?

There is very little literature that explores the difficulties of symptom-recognition in people, like Ben, with severe communication difficulties. In considering symptoms in infants, Selekman and Malloy observed that adult carers subconsciously identified 'cues' (Selekman and Malloy, 1995). This corresponds to the common experience that the recognition of distress seems to be an implicit, rather than explicit, act. Cues have been viewed as 'pieces of information which can be connected together to form patterns' (Thiel *et al*, 1986). This pattern-recognition has been the crucial step missing from much of the work to date on distress in people with severe communication difficulties. In palliative care, this pattern-recognition has been used since 1992 in producing clinical-decision flow diagrams and protocols for communicating with patients with

Table 4.1: Signs and behaviours of distress

Signs	Behaviours
Facial — eg. appearance, tongue movement, jaw movement, eyes.	*Speech* — eg. stuttering, shouting, silence.
Autonomic changes — eg. blood pressure, respiration, pulse rate, skin pallor, sweating.	*Habits and mannerisms* — eg. fidgeting, aggression, agitation, withdrawal, distancing, clinging, food refusal.
Body posture — eg. altered tone, bracing, rubbing.	*Absence of content behaviour* — eg. no longer smiling or making eye-contact.
Vomiting.	
Vocal sounds — eg. moaning, sighing.	

advanced disease, mainly cancer (Regnard and Tempest, 1992; Regnard and Hockley, 1995, 2004). Experience shows that the cues are changes in behaviours and signs, as in *Table 4.1*. These cues appear to be changes from the usual cues observed when the patient is content and carers are able to pick up clues, although they may disagree about their meaning (Porter *et al,* 2001). A major problem is that carers do not routinely document and monitor these cues (Porter *et al,* 2001); consequently, carers are often uncertain about their interpretation.

Several steps in identifying distress can be outlined, which have potential applications in any client or patient unable to communicate effectively, including dementia, severely disabled children, and comatose palliative care patients:

1. A content situation is the one least likely to be associated with distress. It is important to document the signs and behaviour during a content situation if changes are to be noted.
2. Any change away from a content behaviour should be documented, especially as distress may be an absence of content signs and behaviours.
3. These changes should be checked against the signs and behaviours during previous, known episodes of distress eg. constipation, fear of venepuncture.
4. The changes observed and the circumstances in which they occurred can then be checked against clinical-decision checklists.
5. The likeliest cause of the distress is decided, although several possible options may be identified.
6. Treatment of the likeliest cause is started.
7. The signs and behaviours are rechecked. If they have returned to baseline (including content signs and behaviour), then the cause and treatment were correct. If there is no change, then the second on the treatment list (or aother treatment) needs to be tried.

Identifying distress requires knowledge of the patient, knowledge of the population, and knowledge of the science. These three forms of knowledge correspond with those identified by Liaschenko and Fisher (1999), who write about case knowledge (such as pathology); patient knowledge (the individual in the healthcare system); and person knowledge (such as personal biography). This baseline makes it possible to identify a change in behaviour or signs. Three general tools are needed to identify distress:

1. A tool to document the signs and behaviours shown in *Table 4.1*. Baseline observations need to be documented when the client is content, as well as when the client is distressed. The Northgate DisDAT (Disability Distress Assessment Tool) has been developed specifically for this purpose with people with profound communication problems. It differs from previous tools in that it makes no attempt to diagnose the cause of the distress and is not a scoring instrument (Regnard *et al*, 2003). Such documentation tools enable carers to clarify and record observations they already make.
2. A screening-decision checklist (*Panel 4.1*). This enables an initial decision to be made on the general cause of the distress.
3. Specific-decision checklists for specific categories of distress that have been suggested by the screening checklist, such as fear or pain (Regnard and Hockley, 2004). These are used to narrow down general categories of distress to one, or a few, possible causes, which then suggest a specific treatment.

Psychological causes of distress

Ben's story (continued)

The doctor came, he took some blood tests and now he's told the nurses to take me to a hospital where I'll have an operation to remove one of my testicles. Why are they doing this? No-one's told me.

... I've had the operation and I don't feel as sore now, but I'm still feeling unwell. My mum is here — I haven't seen her for a long time. She is crying. My care manager is here too and I heard her tell my mother that I can't go and live with my friends now because I'm too ill. I can't understand why and this makes me sad. I sometimes cry, but when I do the nurses here don't seem to know why; they keep looking at my wound. I don't want people looking at my wound all the time — I want someone to tell me what's happening to me. My mum, the doctors and nurses, they all talk to each other. Why won't anyone talk to me?

The doctor's had a meeting with my family and the other people who work with me and told them that there'd be no more treatment for me. They said something about palliative care, and that it would be best if I went to live in another new hospital. That's worrying and frightening — will the staff there know and understand me?

It can be difficult to interpret the cause of distress. An increase in activity due to distress may be misinterpreted as a challenging behaviour, while reduced activity may be wrongly interpreted as someone being quiet and content. Silence or a reduction in activity as an expression of distress is not surprising when one recognises that suffering often produces loneliness and alienation from others (Younger, 1995). Perhaps not surprisingly, professional carers find it difficult to estimate the patient's ability to communicate (Purcell *et al*, 1999; Porter *et al*, 2001; Banat *et al*, 2002). Carers can view a change in behaviour pessimistically as something that is unlikely to change (Whitehouse *et al*, 2000). Forty percent of people with severe learning disability have challenging behaviours (Ashcroft *et al*, 2001) and up to 45% are on antipsychotics drugs (Ahmed *at al*, 2000;

Panel 4.1: Is the new sign or behaviour:

- **Repeated rapidly?**
Consider: pleuritic pain (in time with breathing)
colic (comes and goes every few minutes)
repetitive movement due to boredom or fear.

- **Associated with breathing?**
Consider: infection
COPD
pleural effusion
cancer.

- **Worsened or precipitated by movement?**
Consider: movement-related pains.

- **Related to eating?**
Consider: food refusal through illness, fear or depression
food refusal because of swallowing problems
upper GI problems (oral hygiene, peptic ulcer, dyspepsia) or abdominal problems.

- **Related to a specific situation?**
Consider: frightening or painful scenarios.

- **Associated with vomiting?**
Consider: causes of nausea and vomiting.

- **Associated with elimination (urine or faecal)?**
Consider: urinary problems (infection, retention)
GI problems (diarrhoea, constipation).

- **Present in a normally comfortable position or situation?**
Consider: pains at rest
infection
nausea.

Ingram, 1991). The situation is further complicated when one realises that the physical symptoms inevitably have a psychological component. Pain, for example, is not simply an unpleasant physical sensation, but is also a distressing experience. It is not just patients who have communication problems because carers have problems understanding their communication!

Despite these difficulties, observant carers may be able intuitively to identify causes of distress when these observations are linked to the context in which they occur. For example, it may be possible to distinguish some of the characteristics of physical symptoms from those of psychological distress (*Table 4.2*).

Claud Regnard, Charlotte L Clarke, Lynn Gibson, Dorothy Matthews

Pain as a cause of distress

Ben's story (continued)

It hurts sometimes when I try to turn over in bed and I get pain in my tummy. The nurses have given me a new bed with a special mattress and they give me medicine for my pain, but my tummy pain is getting worse and sometimes it hurts when I am moved and I shout out loud.

Identifying the cause of pain

Even if pain is suspected, it is essential to identify what type of pain is present since different pains need different treatments.

Are the signs or behaviours of pain related to movement? Pain precipitated by the slightest movement suggests a fracture and this needs to be excluded by an X-ray. Other causes are soft tissue inflammation (eg. bruising due to injury or infection) or joint problems (eg. arthritis). Bone pain due to problems such as bone metastases occur when the bone is strained, such as local pressure or weight bearing. Pain on active movement suggests muscle pain. The commonest muscle pain is myofascial pain, which is precipitated by abnormal use of one muscle (eg. due to abnormal posture) and can cause severe pain on movement. Pain occurring in time with the movements of breathing suggests either a rib problem (eg. fracture or bone metastasis) or pleurisy (eg. infection, pulmonary embolus, or local cancer). Chest pain associated with exercise suggests angina due to coronary artery disease.

Are the signs or behaviours of pain periodic? Pain that regularly occurs every few seconds is likely to be related to breathing and causes include the rib and pleuritic problems mentioned in the section above. Pain that occurs every few minutes is likely to be colic. This is most commonly bowel colic (usually due to constipation), but can also be caused by colic of the bladder (eg. urinary tract infection), uterus (eg. period pain), gallbladder (eg, cholecystitis) or ureter (eg. renal stones or ureteric obstruction by cancer).

Are the signs and behaviours of pain related to a procedure? Even familiar procedures can be painful, such as taking blood or changing dressings.

Are the signs and behaviours of pain related to eating? This may be caused by pain in the mouth (eg. dental problems, mucosal infection, cancer), in the pharynx or oesophagus (eg. mucosal infection, cancer, acid reflux), or the stomach and duodenum (eg. gastritis, peptic ulceration or cancer). The commonest mucosal infection is due to the yeast candida.

Table 4.2: Distinguishing physical causes from psychological ones

Feature	Physical causes	Psychological causes
Context	Related to physical context eg. movement, elimination, breathing, uncomfortable or painful procedure.	Frightening situations, eg. hospital visit. Unfamiliar situations.
Signs	No specific signs.	No specific signs.
Behaviours	Adaptive, eg. rubbing or holding a painful area, keeping an area still. Food refusal due to loss of appetite. Distractive, eg. rocking (or other rhythmic movements), pacing, biting hand or lip, gesturing, clenched fists.	Reduced activity and responses are more likely in depression, and increased activity is more likely in anger or anxiety. NB. anxiety or depression may accompany physical symptoms. Avoidance of frightening situations.
Examples	Nausea: pale, food refusal, vomiting, reduced pulse rate. Fractured wrist: holding wrist, refusing to use that hand. Constipation: regular signs or behaviours of distress every few minutes.	Depression: withdrawn, quiet, reduced responses, reduced appetite or food refusal, constipation. Anxiety: agitated, sweating, dilated pupils, increased pulse rate, reduced appetite or food refusal. Anger: features of anxiety with frustration and refusal to cooperate.

Are the signs and behaviours of pain worsened by passing stool or urine? The commonest cause of pain on micturition is a urinary tract infection, but pain can also be caused by catheters or the presence of local cancer. A hard stool due to constipation is the commonest cause of pain on defaecation, but other causes include anal fissures, haemorrhoids and local cancer.

Are there any associated skin changes in the area of the pain? Skin ulcers are often painful and can be caused by problems such as local pressure damage, skin disease (eg. dermatitis, psoriasis), local cancer, or vascular problems (arterial insufficiency or venous incompetence).

Are the signs or behaviours of pain associated with altered sensation? When pain is suspected in an area of the body, any increased response to touch (hypersensitivity) or pain on touching (allodynia) in that same area suggests the presence of neuropathic pain. Such pains are precipitated by nerve damage and persist long after the cause of the damage has gone. An example is the neuralgia seen after a herpes zoster infection where pain can persist for years, even though the infection healed after a few weeks. Pain in an area of reduced sensation may be due to nerve compression such as sciatica.

Are the signs or behaviours of pain persisting? Pain can persist because of unresolved fear, misunderstanding or depression. It will also persist if the medication is being given too infrequently; the dose is too low; or the preparation is unpleasant or difficult to take. Finally, persisting pain can be due to the onset of a new pain. Advice from a pain or palliative care specialist can be helpful when pain persists in spite of assessment and treatment.

Managing pain

Once an assessment of the pain has been made, it is usually possible to narrow down the likely cause to one or two choices. Which treatment is used is entirely dependent on the likely cause, since there is no single treatment that treats all pains. Attempting to treat all pains with the same analgesic will often result in failure or adverse effects. For example, the pain of abdominal colic can be worsened by opioids such as codeine or morphine. Other pains need drugs such as corticosteroids which reduce the swelling around tumours and reduce the pressure on surrounding nerves, or some anticonvulsants and tricyclics which are used to treat neuropathic pain such as the neuralgia occurring after zoster shingles infection. Some pains do not need drug treatment at all — for example, myofascial pain which can cause troublesome pain on movement and yet is rapidly treated with the application of a transcutaneous electrical nerve stimulator (TENS) or acupuncture. *Table 4.3* is a summary of first line treatments for different pains.

Understanding analgesics

Primary and secondary analgesics: most commonly used analgesics have a direct action on blocking pain pathways. These are the primary analgesics and include non-opioids (eg. paracetamol), weak opioids (eg. codeine) and strong opioids (eg. morphine). It is common to start with paracetamol, move to codeine if this is ineffective, and then move to morphine if the pain persists. Other drugs can relieve pain through an indirect mechanism. These are the secondary analgesics, also called co-analgesics or adjuvant analgesics. Examples include hyoscine butylbromide for colic, amitriptyline for neuropathic pain, and dexamethasone for nerve-compression pain due to tumour. It is common to use primary and secondary analgesics together. If pain is frequent or continuous, the analgesic should be prescribed regularly, since using them on an 'as required' basis results in poor pain relief — continuous pain needs continuous analgesia.

Strong opioids: there is much ignorance and misunderstanding around strong opioids, such as morphine. In reality, these are effective analgesics that are safe when used correctly (see below for adverse effects). Most strong opioids are equally effective — ie. they treat the same range of pains. Some strong opioids are more potent than others — ie. less of the drug is needed to have the

Table 4.3: Different treatments according to types of pain (for more information, see Regnard and Hockley, 2003)

Pain	Features	First line management
Bone pain due to metastases or osteoporosis.	Pain on weight bearing or straining the affected bone.	Find positions and activities that are least painful. Refer to pain or palliative care teams for advice on strong opioids and the use of bisphosphonates. Radiotherapy can reduce pain in 65% of patients with bone metastases.
Colic	Regular pain occurring every few minutes.	Treat the cause, eg: –abdominal colic: treat constipation. –urinary colic: exclude urinary tract infection or renal stones. If persistent (eg. bowel obstruction due to cancer) refer to palliative care team for advice on the use of hyoscine butylbromide.
Eating-related pain	Food refusal, pain during eating or swallowing, abdominal pain.	Exclude dental problems or oral infection (candida, herpes simplex or zoster) and refer for treatment. Refer for medical opinion for assessing oesophageal and gastric causes. An antacid may help as a temporary measure.
Elimination-related pain	Pain on passing urine or stool.	Constipation: adjust laxatives to produce a comfortable stool without colic. Urinary tract infection: culture urine and treat. Haemorrhoids: use local cream. Local cancer: refer to palliative care team for advice.
Exercise chest pain	Tightness or heaviness in chest, perhaps with breathlessness.	Refer for medical opinion to exclude angina.
Fracture	Pain on the slightest passive movement.	Referral for X-ray and assessment.

Table 4.3: Different treatments according to types of pain (for more information, see Regnard and Hockley, 2003)

Joint pain	Pain on moving joint, sometimes with local swelling.	Refer for medical opinion to assess cause. Paracetamol 1g 4-6 hourly may help, but NSAIDs may be needed.
Myofascial pain	Pain on using affected muscle with local tenderness in the muscle.	Local cooling may help. Ask for advice on the use of a TENS, otherwise refer to pain or palliative care team for assessment.
Neuropathic pain	Sensitivity or pain on light touch.	Refer to pain or palliative care team for advice on the use of amitriptyline or gabapentin.
Persisting pain	Pain persisting despite treatment.	Exclude anxiety, anger or depression. Refer to pain or palliative care team for advice.
Procedure pain	Pain due to a specific procedure.	Modify procedure eg. use local anaesthetic cream prior to taking a blood sample.
Skin inflammation	Redness, ulceration or weeping of skin.	Refer for medical opinion to assess cause. Pressure ulcer: institute local pressure care and pressure ulcer policy. Malignant ulcer: refer to palliative care team for advice.
Soft tissue injury	Visible bruising, local pain on pressure.	Exclude serious injury. Local cooling may help. If still painful try paracetamol 1g 4-6 hourly.

same effect, but this does not make them more effective. For example, fentanyl is nearly 150 times more potent than morphine, but it treats the same range of pains. By contrast, methadone is similar in potency to morphine, but can be more effective for some pains, such as neuropathic pain.

All opioids are deactivated in the liver with the exception of morphine, which is converted to potent, active metabolites that are excreted through the kidney. The result is that liver disease has only a modest effect on the patient's ability to handle morphine, but any change in kidney function causes the active metabolites to accumulate. By contrast, most strong opioids are more affected by liver disease, but less affected by kidney disease.

The median daily dose of oral morphine is 100mg, but the final required dose of a strong opioid cannot be predicted by assessing weight, age, sex or surface area. Consequently, patients are started on low doses that are gradually increased (usually in 25–50% steps every two to three days) until the patient is comfortable. Very few patients need more than 500mg daily.

Adverse effects of analgesics: problems with paracetamol are unusual as long as doses are not higher than 1g four-hourly. By contrast, gastric irritation is common with non-steroidal anti-inflammatory (NSAID) drugs and can cause severe bleeding from the gut, although this is less of a problem with NSAID drugs such as ibuprofen. However, all NSAIDs can cause renal damage, especially if the patient is dehydrated.

Addiction is not seen in patients taking strong opioids for pain relief (Passik and Portenoy, 1998; Borgbjerg *et al*, 1996). The beneficial effect of strong opioids on pain does not wear off, and drug doses do not have to be repeatedly escalated (Taub, 1982). There is no evidence that strong opioids either hasten death or shorten life (Regnard and Badger, 1987; Cools *et al*, 1996; Twycross and Wilcock, 2001). Most patients are not troubled with adverse effects since, unlike analgesia, tolerance to most adverse effects does occur. For example, mild drowsiness wears off within a few days, while tolerance to respiratory depression is so rapid that respiratory depression is rare in routine use of strong opioids. One exception is that, like analgesia, constipation does not wear off, and nearly all patients on weak or strong opioids should be prescribed a laxative. If adverse effects are a problem, there are now effective alternative strong opioids that can be used, such as hydromorphone, oxycodone and fentanyl.

Constipation, nausea and vomiting

Ben's story (continued)

Lots of different people have been to see me and examine me this week. I heard them tell my mother they were assessing me; I don't know what for! I've joined in some sessions, including moving to music and being in a water pool, which was very relaxing. It hurts when I go to the toilet and I've been sick. The staff want me to eat my meals, but I don't want to.

In advanced disease, it is common to eat less, which results in a reduced frequency of bowel motions. Consequently, frequency of passing stool cannot be used as a definition of constipation. By contrast, a hard stool that is uncomfortable to pass suggests constipation. Causes include reduced intake of fibre, reduced fluid intake, drugs that slow the bowel such as analgesics, causes of dehydration and anything that makes passing stool painful, such as local tumour or haemorrhoids.

The management of constipation is detailed in *Panel 4.2*. If no stool has been passed at all for more than five days, then bowel obstruction needs to be excluded. For causes of constipation, the correct choice of laxatives is important. Mild constipation can be treated with a gentle laxative,

**Panel 4.2: Clinical decisions for managing constipation
(for further information see Regnard and Hockley, 2003)**

1. Is this bowel obstruction? — Refer for a surgical opinion.
2. Is there a treatable cause? — Correct dehydration or change to less constipating drugs.
3. Ensure privacy.
4. Is this mild constipation? — Use a gentle laxative, eg. docusate.
5. Is the rectum or stoma full? — Start stimulant and softening laxatives, eg. senna and docusate.
6. Is the constipation persisting? — Exclude local rectal problems, eg. haemorrhoids; consider Movicol.

such as docusate. Low doses of lactulose such as 5–10mls twelve-hourly can be used as an alternative, but higher doses commonly cause abdominal bloating and discomfort. Moderate to severe constipation often needs a combination of a stimulant laxative (senna or bisacodyl) and a softening laxative, such as docusate or low-dose lactulose. Dantron is a stimulant laxative that is available in commercial combinations, but these tend to be expensive and dantron has problems such as colouring the urine red (giving the impression of bleeding) and can cause chemical burns around the anus. For patients with hard stool in the large bowel, Movicol is a laxative that, when mixed with water (125mls plus one sachet), can help soften and clear impacted stool. Hard stool in the rectum may clear with a suppository, but occasionally a manual evacuation is needed, which is best done under mild sedation.

Treatments of nausea and vomiting are summarised in *Panel 4.3*. If vomiting is present, immediate measures include a large bowl, tissues and water to rinse out the mouth. If the problem is mainly vomiting, it may be gastric stasis due to poor gastric emptying, and this responds to drugs that encourage normal gastric emptying, such as domperidone or metoclopramide. Other causes of vomiting with little or no nausea include oesophageal obstruction or raised intracranial pressure, but these are much less common. Nausea (with or without vomiting) has many causes. Biochemical causes (drugs, hypercalcaemia, bacterial toxins) will often respond to low doses

**Panel 4.3: Clinical decisions in managing nausea and vomiting
(for further information see Regnard and Hockley, 2003)**

1. If vomiting, make available a large bowl, tissues and water.
2. Is the patient troubled mainly by vomiting? Consider gastric stasis — start metoclopramide or domperidone, 10–20mg 8–hourly.
3. Could the cause be drugs, toxins or biochemical? Start haloperidol 1.5–3mg at bedtime.
4. Is the nausea or vomiting worse on movement? Exclude an ear infection or travel sickness.
5. Is gastritis present? Stop drugs causing gastritis. Start a proton pump inhibitor, eg. omeprazole.
6. Could fear or anxiety be contributing? Find the cause and provide support.
7. Is the nausea or vomiting persisting? Start cyclizine 25–50mg 8–hourly or levomepromazine 5–12.5mg at bedtime.

NB. Metoclopramide, haloperidol and levomepromazine can all be given subcutaneously; domperidone can be given rectally.

of haloperidol (1.5–3mg once at night). If the nausea or vomiting are related to movement, an ear infection needs to be excluded. Other causes of nausea or vomiting include gastric irritation (NSAIDs, steroids, anxiety) and the effects of fear or anxiety. Persistent nausea or vomiting in advanced disease may respond to cyclizine or levomepromazine. Many antiemetics need to be given by parenteral routes initially. Metoclopramide, haloperidol and levomepromazine can all be give subcutaneously, while domperidone can be given rectally.

Answering difficult questions

Ben's story (continued)

Sometimes when the nurses are washing or dressing me, it hurts a lot and I shout. I don't like it when I am on my own — it makes me upset and anxious. I don't know what's happening to me; I'm frightened. I ask the nurses, but they talk about other things and won't tell me. I'm meeting lots of new people and I'm getting to know them better, but I don't know whether they know me. What does it mean, 'having cancer'? It must be bad news if my mother is crying.

An overview of difficult questions is in *Panel 4.4*. Such questions are very important. They may be asked by the patient or their family and arise out of a person's uncertainty as they struggle to adjust to their changing circumstances. The importance of these questions lies in the role they play in helping the person to adjust, but they often arise at a time where the future is unclear. Consequently:

- acknowledging the question is important
- answers may be unclear or impossible
- some answers will require the breaking of bad news.

Difficult questions are often asked spontaneously, so that the setting is not always ideal, but the person may have chosen that setting because they feel safe to ask in that situation. It is helpful to check what the person means by the question — for example, asking 'How much time is left?' may have nothing to do with dying and everything to do with the time for lunch! Despite acknowledging and checking a difficult question, a clear answer may be impossible because there is insufficient information available. Being honest about not knowing improves, rather than hinders, a relationship. If the question is impossible to answer because the professional carer does not have the experience or knowledge, then the patients needs to be referred to someone who does. In many cases, an answer is possible, but this means breaking bad news.

Bad news is always bad, but it does not have to be told badly. The first step is to check whether the person is able to understand new information and in what form they would prefer that information. Then it is important to find out how much the person already knows and whether they want to know more. If they want more information, it is essential to provide some form of

> **Panel 4.4: Clinical decisions in answering difficult questions and breaking bad news (for further information see Regnard and Hockley, 2003)**
>
> 1. Acknowledge the importance of the question.
> 2. Is the setting appropriate? Either accept the setting or suggest moving elsewhere.
> 3. Check why the question is being asked.
> 4. Is a clear answer difficult or impossible? If this is due to inexperience or lack of knowledge, refer to someone who has this. If a clear answer is impossible, then be honest about not knowing the answer.
> 5. If the answer is bad news: check if the person is able to understand and in what form they would prefer the information. Check what they know now and whether they want to know more. Warn — let them know that you have some bad news, eg. 'The tests were abnormal'. Pause — observe the reaction to the warning. Check if they want you to continue, eg. 'Do you want to me to explain what is wrong?' Continue at the patient's pace — not at the professional's.

warning that bad news is coming. This may be sitting the person down with a cup of tea, or saying, 'It's not good news'. A pause allows the professional to observe the reaction, followed by a check to ask if they what more information. Most people make it clear whether they do or do not want to know; occasionally, some people are uncertain because they need more time, which needs to be acknowledged and rechecked at a later stage. The key to breaking bad news is to do it at the person's pace — not the professional's. It is never the role of a professional to decide whether a patient should be told, but to find out what the patient *wants* to know.

Breathing problems

Ben's story (continued)

My mother is happier this week; she has been to see the vicar who came to see me. At first, she didn't want to see him or the Macmillan nurse, I think she's called, but I'm happier because she is! I know that I am not so well because I just want to sleep most of the time, and when I am awake I can't get out of bed any more. Sometimes, I cannot breathe properly; the nurse said I was more breathless and put a mask on my face, which helped. My chest sounds terrible; I rattle when I breathe and when I try to cough it doesn't work very well, so the nurses help me by using a suction machine to clear my mouth.

Breathlessness is common in advanced disease. Any sudden or severe breathlessness needs an urgent assessment and may need admission to hospital, since some causes can be treated and reversed. Simple measures can ease the sensation of breathlessness and can be started by any carer (*Panel 4.5*). If a chest infection is the cause of the breathlessness, then treatment is appropriate. There is no ethical difficulty here since the infection is causing distressing problems and an antibiotic is the simplest and quickest way to relieve that distress.

Breathlessness is often accompanied by fear, which can be helped by the simple measures in *Panel 4.5*, but occasionally this is severe and may need medication. Opioids can help breathlessness

> **Panel 4.5: Simple measures for breathlessness that can be started by any carer**
>
> 1. Call for help.
> 2. Sit the patient upright.
> 3. Increase air movement over the patient's face (a gentle fan or opening a window will do this).
> 4. Help the patient relax the shoulders by massaging them in a downwards direction (this reverses the 'hunching' caused by anxiety and increases the capacity to breathe).
> 5. Explain what is happening and stay with the patient.

and are titrated the same way as for pain (Boyd and Kelly, 1997; Flowers, 2003). Lorazepam 0.5-1mg orally provides relaxation with minimal sedation. More severe and persistent breathlessness in a patient who is remaining at home needs the advice of a palliative care physician.

The last hours and days

Ben's story (continued)

I am happy that people sit with me, even when they think I am asleep. I feel calmer when people are with me; I think it's because I am not so frightened. I am very tired now and lie with my eyes shut most of the time. My mother insists on playing soppy music but I don't want that I want my rock music, I am not able to control what is happening to me any more so why won't she let me choose my own music? If I could just throw that cup to let her know I hate soppy tunes.

I am very comfortable now — maybe my mother's got the message, at last she's put some decent rock music. I think that I will just go to sleep.

Diagnosing the onset of the dying phase is harder for some teams than others, but there are signs and behaviours that suggest a patient has entered the last hours and days (*Panel 4.6*). If the team is clear that this is the situation, then a number of goals need to be achieved (*Panel 4.7*). Following these goals will help most patients, but if the treatments are unhelpful or cannot be used, it is important to contact the local palliative care team for advice. Since the patient is dying naturally of their disease, resuscitation would be of no benefit to the patient; consequently, there is no resuscitation decision to be made — only a 'Do Not Attempt Resuscitation' order to be documented (Regnard and Randall, 2005). This means that relatives do not have to be asked for permission not to resuscitate, but they must be kept informed of developments, as in goals seven to eleven of the Care Pathway for the Dying Patient (*Panel 4.7*). In most cases, a patient will die comfortably and peacefully; it will be more a gentle 'winding down' than any sudden presence of death.

Claud Regnard, Charlotte L Clarke, Lynn Gibson, Dorothy Matthews

---

Panel 4.6: Signs and behaviours that suggest a patient is dying
(Regnard and Hockley, 2003)

- Deteriorating day by day or faster because of the underlying condition, or an irreversible complication of their disease.
- Patient expresses a realisation that he or she is dying.
- Reduced cognition; patient drowsy or comatose.
- Bed-bound.
- Taking little food or fluid and having difficulty with oral medication.
- Altered breathing pattern.
- Peripherally cyanosed and cold.

Panel 4.7: Goals in the Care Pathway for the Dying Patient
(adapted from Ellershaw and Ward, 2003)

1. Current medication is assessed and non-essentials discontinued. Stop all non-essential medication and if unable to swallow convert to SC route or once-daily preparations.
2. As required subcutaneous medication written up as follows:
Pain:

if not on oral morphine, use or prescribe diamorphine 2.5mg SC 4–hourly PRN.

if already on morphine, convert to a diamorphine SC infusion (ask palliative care team for advice on conversions).
Nausea and vomiting:

use or prescribe cyclizine 25–50mg SC 8–hourly PRN.
Respiratory-tract secretions:

use or prescribe hyoscine hydrobromide 400microg. SC 8–hourly PRN.
Terminal restlessness and agitation:

use or prescribe midazolam 5–10mg SC 1–2 hourly PRN.
3. Discontinue inappropriate interventions, eg. regular blood tests.
4. Assess the ability to communicate in English.
5. Assess the patient's insight into their condition.
6. Assess the religious and spiritual needs.
7. Identify how the family and others are to be informed of the patient's impending death.
8. Give family and other relevant people the information they need.
9. Ensure that all the key people are aware of the patient's condition.
10. Discuss and explain the plan of care with the patient and family.
11. Ensure that the family and other people involved express an understanding of the plan of care.

Conclusion

There are two key messages that we would like readers to take from this chapter, and which are critical to the management of distress for someone like Ben, who has a learning disability and palliative care needs.

The first message is that there is a need to be able to identify and assess the person's distress. This requires sensitivity to the individual as well as an awareness of the ways of managing need. This sensitivity can be magnified by ensuring that staff know the patients they work with, and that the services are organised in a way that allows them sustained contact with the person over a period of time. This sensitivity to distress-recognition may be augmented through the use of an assessment mechanism such as DISDAT (Regnard *et al*, 2003).

The second message is that there is a persistence of therapeutic intent that does not waver, even when someone is facing his or her last days. The therapeutic intent is always there with the purpose of acting to alleviate distress. Much can be achieved through symptom management, but much too can be achieved by ensuring not just excellent physical care, but also that the needs of the whole person are met. This can only take place through the relationship that staff and family members have with the individual. The therapeutic intent of palliative care requires also that a great deal of attention is paid to developing interventions and interactions with people. Davis and Sheldon (1997), for example, highlight the developing simultaneous use of pharmacological and non-pharmacological interventions and increasing use of complementary therapies.

Our final thoughts must turn to Ben and his mother. Our unending challenge to ourselves must be to ensure that a learning disability and the palliative care needs of a person do not obscure and obstruct our ability to identify and meet those needs.

References

Ahmed Z, Fraser W, Kerr MP, *et al* (2000) Reducing antipsychotic education in people with learning disability. *Br J Psychiatry* **176**: 42–6

Ashcroft R, Fraser B, Kerr M, Ahmed Z (2001) Are antipsychotic drugs the right treatment for challenging behaviour in learning disability?: the lace of a randomised trial. *J Med Ethics* **27**: 338–43

Banat D, Summers S, Pring T (2002) An investigation into carers' perceptions of the verbal comprehension ability of adults with severe learning disabilities. *Br J Develop Disabil* **30**: 78–81

Borgbjerg FM, Nielsen K, Franks J (1996) Experimental pain stimulates respiration and attenuates morphine-induced respiratory depression: a controlled study in human volunteers. *Pain* **64**(1): 123–8

Boyd KJ, Kelly M (1997) Oral morphine as symptomatic treatment of dyspnoea in patients with advanced cancer. *Palliat Med* **11**(4): 277–81

Cools HJ, Berkhout AM, De Bock GH (1996) Subcutaneous morphine infusion by syringe drivers for terminally ill patients. *Age Ageing* **25**(3): 206–8

Corner J, Dunlop R (1997) New approaches to care. In: Clarke D, Hockley J, Ahmedzai S (eds) (1997) *New Themes in Palliative Care*. Open University Press, Berkshire

Davis CL, Sheldon F (1997) Therapeutic innovations. In: Clarke D, Hockley J, Ahmedzai S (eds) (1997) *New Themes in Palliative Care*. Open University Press, Berkshire

Ellershaw J, Ward C (2003) Care of the dying patient: the last hours and days of life. *BMJ* **326**: 30–4

Flowers B (2003) Palliative care for patients with end-stage heart failure. *Nurs Times* **99**: 30–2

George R, Sykes J (1997) Beyond cancer? In: Clarke D, Hockley J, Ahmedzai S (eds) (1997) *New Themes in Palliative Care*. Open University Press, Berkshire

Ingram R (1991) Learning difficulties and communication. *Nurs Stand* **5**: 36–9

Liaschenko J, Fisher A (1999) Theorizing the knowledge that nurses use in the conduct of their work. *Sch Inq Nurs Pract* **13**: 29–41

Passik S, Portenoy R (1998) Substance abuse issues in palliative care. In: Berger A (ed) (1998) *Principles and Practice of Supportive Oncology*. Lippincott-Raven, Philadephia

Porter J, Ouvry C, Morgan M, Downs C (2001) Interpreting the communication of people with profound and multiple learning difficulties. *Br J Learn Disabil* **29**: 12–16

Purcell M, Morris I, McConkey R (1999) Staff perceptions of the communicative competence of adult persons with intellectual disabilities. *Br J Develop Disabil* **45**: 16–25

Regnard C, Badger C (1987) Opioids, sleep and the time of death. *Palliat Med* **1**(2): 107–10

Regnard C, Tempest S (1992) *A Guide to Symptom Relief in Advanced Cancer*. 3rd edn. Haigh and Hochland, Manchester

Regnard C, Hockley J (eds) (1995) *Flow Diagrams in Advanced Cancer and other Diseases*. Edward Arnold, London

Regnard C, Hockley J (2004) *Guide to Symptom Relief in Palliative Care*. 5th edn. Radcliffe, Abingdon

Regnard C, Matthews D, Gibson L, Clarke C, Watson B (2003) Difficulties in identifying distress and its causes in people with severe communication problems. *Int J Palliat Nurs* **9**(3): 173–6

Regnard C, Randall F (2005) A framework for making advance decisions on resuscitation. *Clin Med* **5**(4): 354–60

Selekman J, Malloy E (1995) Difficulties in symptom recognition in infants. *J Paediat Nurs* **10**: 89–92

Taub A (1982) Opioid analgesics in the treatment of chronic intractable pain of non-neoplastic origin. In: Kitahata LM, Collins JG (eds) (1982) *Narcotic Analgesics in Anaesthesiology*. Williams and Watkins, Baltimore

Thiel J, Baltwin J, Hyde R, Sloan B, Strandquist G (1986) An investigation of decision theory: what are the effects of teaching cue recognition? *J Nurs Educ* **25**: 319–24

Twycross R, Wilcock (2001) Pain relief. In: *Symptom Management in Advanced Cancer*. Radcliffe, Abingdon

Whitehouse R, Chamberlain P, Tunna K (2000) Dementia in people with learning disability: a preliminary study into care staff knowledge and attributions. *Br J Learn Disabil* **28**: 148–53

Younger J (1995) The alienation of the sufferer. *Adv Nurs Sci* **17**: 53–72

CHAPTER 5

The role of the learning-disability nurse — meeting individual needs

Siri Persaud

Learning-disability nurses (LDNs) work in a variety of settings, including residential care (hospital and community), day care facilities, assessment and treatment units and community-based resources (CLDTs). Whatever settings they work in, they aim to support people with learning disabilities to live full and independent lives in the community. Their work often involves the individuals, their families, carers (paid or unpaid), other professionals and independent agencies (eg. Mencap).

There is much evidence that people with learning disabilities are now living longer and experiencing the same health problems as the rest of the non-disabled population. It is also recognised that such individuals will need resources to meet those health needs and will need palliative care for those illnesses that are non-responsive to curative treatment. In the context of the latter, there is an important role to be played by the LDN.

This chapter aims to identify the key roles and responsibilities of the LDN when accessing palliative care services for people with learning disabilities.

Roles and responsibilities

The last few decades have seen the closures of large institutions and the resettlement of people with learning disabilities in the community (DoH, 1971). The large hospitals not only provided a home, but were also the main source by which the health needs of the people who resided there were met (DoH, 1998). Living in the community means that there are not many different ways to meet the ongoing health needs of this population. As a result, there is much more use of generic health services and people with learning disabilities now depend on primary health care services too (DoH, 2001), as do many non-disabled people. Nevertheless, their health needs are often overlooked and people with learning disabilities face inequalities in health care provision (Mencap, 1998). Although some achievements have been made since the 1971 Government White Paper *Better Services for the Mentally Handicapped*, it is acknowledged that the health care needs of people with learning disabilities often go unmet (Mencap, 1998; DoH, 1998). Illnesses and premature death can be avoided, and more work needs to be done to improve access to mainstream health services (Tuffrey-Wijne, 1997; Howells, 1997; Sperlinger and O'Hara, 1997; DoH, 1998; Read, 1998).

The number of people with learning disabilities is estimated to increase (Mencap, 1998) and is an indication that they are now living longer and having increasing health needs (Jancar, 1988). This places more demands on primary and community health resources, due to additional and potential physical illnesses, in addition to their learning disability. It is recognised that, for example, people with Down syndrome may also have increased risks of cardiovascular diseases, respiratory illness, Alzheimer's disease, leukaemia and hypothyroidism (Lott and McCoy, 1992). Similarly, to the non-disabled population, people with learning disability are also affected by physical illnesses such as cancer, multiple sclerosis, cardiopulmonary diseases, and renal failure (DoH 1995; Jancar and Jancar 1977; Stanley 1998). These illnesses in particular may require palliative care services.

Nurses are often the primary care giver to many people with learning disabilities and their role within the palliative care setting may be pivotal and varied.

Building on what's gone before

The role of the LDN has been in contention for a number of years. Since the 1970s (and probably at the beginning of the twentieth century), several documents criticised learning disability hospital care and debated whether LDNs should work under a health, medical or social model (Briggs, 1972; DoH, 1995; Jay, 1979; Beacock, 1999; Alaszewski *et al*, 2001; Boarder, 2002). As people with learning disabilities were resettled within the community, learning disability nursing was becoming more community-orientated (Boarder, 2002). Nurses were, therefore, in a pivotal position to provide support and advice to both the medical services (including primary healthcare services) and the client. During a time when the role of the nurse was perceived as important in the health context within the community, education grew, which was reflected in the development and implementation of the Project 2000 nursing curriculum (Boarder, 2002). This was assisted by the learning disability project in 1995, Continuing the Commitment, which focused the role of the LDN in the direction of health — ie. health promotion, health care, health surveillance (Kay *et al*, 1995). This pathway has also been emphasised in Government initiatives such as *Signposts for Success* (DoH, 1998) and *Valuing People: a Strategy for Learning Disability for the 21st Century* (DoH, 2001). These documents have highlighted the difficulties and problems people with learning disabilities face when accessing generic services to meet their health needs. They also assert that LDNs need to revisit their roles and adapt their skills to meet the new challenges ahead.

LDNs have drawn their skills and experiences from rich sources, such as specialised pre-registration education leading to Registered Nurse Mental Handicap (RNMH) or what is now known as Registered Nurse Learning Disabilities (RNLD); medicine; society generally; and, most importantly, from people with learning disabilities themselves and their associated carers. This can put them on a firm foundation to deliver and coordinate high-quality health care for the individual who has health needs.

The Royal College of Nursing (RCN, 2003) has produced a definition of nursing:

The use of clinical judgement in the provision of care to enable people to improve, maintain, or recover health to cope with health problems, and to achieve the best possible quality of life, whatever their disease or disability until death.

This definition could not have appeared at a better time. It helps nurses to explain their values, define themselves and what they do, and is applicable to every field of nursing. If, as nurses, we cannot define what we do, we cannot measure it; if we cannot measure it, we cannot evaluate it; and if we cannot evaluate it, we cannot improve it.

It is difficult to define learning disability nursing clearly. This may be due to the ongoing changes and diverse ways that LDNs are practicing (Boarder, 2002). However, Kay *et al* (1995) suggest that learning disability nursing could be described as assessing, providing and evaluating the support, which contributes to bringing about the optimal health status of the person with a learning disability. This intervention seeks to improve and maintain the health and way of life of this population.

Using a case study approach

The following three case studies will help highlight the role of the LDN and illustrate the diverse nature of this role in the palliative care setting. Each one is different in its own way. All names have been changed for the purpose of confidentiality.

Case Study One

Name: Josh.
Age: 21.
Diagnosis: Down syndrome; diabetes; heart defect; cyanotic attacks.
Prognosis: No formal prognosis of life expectancy.

Background

This twenty-one year-old man lived at home with his mother, and had come to live in the UK in the early 1990s after she moved here from a non-English-speaking country. His father decided to leave when he was born, leaving his mother to raise and care for him. Due to his illnesses, Josh missed out on his education, both at special-school and further-education levels.

Behaviourally, Josh is able to manipulate various situations and demands his mother's attention by refusing to eat certain foods or eat regularly. He tends to monopolise his mother; interrupts when his mother is in conversation with her current husband; and will not speak English when his paid carer is present. On occasion, he will insist he is going to leave home and get married. His difficult behaviour extends to not complying with routines and not responding when spoken to.

Medical background

Josh was diagnosed as having Down syndrome with a congenital heart defect and diabetes. The diabetes is controlled by diet and insulin, which is managed by his mother. He needs blood tests before insulin is administered by injection, and each time he has a cyanotic attack he requires medical attention for oxygen therapy and morphine (orally and by injection), which is administered by his mother. A strict care plan is followed for this procedure, and if it fails, hospital admission is usually necessary for further such intervention. This caused much stress, anxiety and fear, both for the family and Josh. Prognosis is poor, but there is no set time given and this has caused difficulty when accessing hospice services.

Josh's understanding of his condition

Nobody can be sure how much understanding Josh has of his conditions. He is evidently frightened every time he has an attack and is always fearful of another. He is aware, owing to his tiredness, that his diabetes makes him unwell. His conditions make it difficult for him to walk long distances, so he uses a wheelchair. Additionally, he suffers regular bouts of breathlessness, leaving his extremities blue due to poor circulation. Although his mother is aware of the short life expectancy, she provides excellent care and acknowledges that her son's physical conditions are deteriorating.

Agencies involved

Health Care Assistants from a nursing agency visit once weekly to provide support by helping get Josh out of bed in the morning, and undertake some personal hygiene tasks. Josh also has input from the District Nursing Service, which involves infrequent visits with a variety of nurses, which Josh finds difficult. Josh takes a long time to get to know and trust someone. The District Nurses formulated nursing care plans for hospice at home nurses. They will not administer emergency intra-muscular injection (morphine) without the GP being present, who often refused to be called out. Josh also uses the Hospice At Home service, which provides one day per week respite for his parents.

Following discharge from the children's hospital, the only contact the GP has had was for ongoing repeat prescription without seeing Josh to review his medication. The GP did not agree with the care plan and would therefore not prescribe morphine for pain-management. He viewed Josh's condition as 'not terminally ill', but his illness will have serious consequences at any time, which would need palliative care services.

Effects of his condition

Due to his age, Josh has recently gone through the transition stage from children to adult services, so respite care at the children's hospice is no longer an option. His care is now under adult cardiac services. His condition prevents him from living life as a twenty-one year-old young man. He is unable to access day services as there are none available to meet the complexity of his needs, and learning disability services are unable to manage his health needs either (ie. medical intervention, respite services, emergency treatment). The hospice is difficult to access because of his learning-disability needs, his age and, ultimately, his non-diagnosis of a 'terminal illness'.

LDN involvement

The LDN supports family and professionals by liaising and offering advice on behaviour management. Input also involved coordinating services, arranging regular reviews, and developing care plans to meet Josh's healthcare needs.

This case demonstrates well the difficulty that someone with a learning disability has in accessing palliative care services. It shows the complexities of needs and the resultant challenges posed to the healthcare team. It is important that the LDN gains the trust and confidence of the individual, whether they live at home (with their family) or in a residential setting (hospital or shared accommodation). In this situation, the LDN should be able to:

1. Assess the needs of the individual, and develop care plans demonstrating the intervention of each of the professionals' individual services.
2. Coordinate the individual's care by organising care reviews that will involve the individual and their family (if this is their choice) and each relevant professional, including primary health care service and palliative care service.
3. Maintain regular appointments, which will include home visits, GP, and clinic appointments so that progress is explained and communicated to the individual and other professionals.
4. Refer on to other appropriate agencies to access services — eg. social events, activities, holidays, which are non-health-related, but may have a positive effect on the health and quality of life of the individual (and their family/carer).
5. Provide training, education and health promotion for the individual to explain and enable awareness of their illness — and also for other professionals to make them aware of learning-disability issues and behaviour management in order to increase their awareness of previous illness and available resources.
6. Develop pathways to affect emergency admission.
7. Although palliative care services were able to offer some input to Josh's care, there was no formal agreement with the learning-disability service to work collaboratively to develop packages of care. This is an area where a formal framework for collaborative working is developed and agreed and will aid a proactive, rather than reactive, approach to care. The LDN could coordinate this framework.
8. Act as an advocate for health needs, and identify how these needs can be best met.
9. Be a coordinator among the various services and agencies involved, and liaise closely to enable effective communication.

In a case like this, the LDN should be able to develop and commission appropriate packages of care to meet the changing and complex needs of the person with learning disabilities. This client group should be able to access palliative care services without prejudice against their age or learning disabilities. The *NHS Cancer Plan* (NHS, 2000) makes specific reference to the needs of cancer patients, ensuring that they have appropriate advice on screening and lifestyle, and access to cancer services. This applies equally to people with learning disabilities who have particular requirements.

Case Study Two

Name: Donald.
Age: 27.
Diagnosis: Learning disability (moderate); severe epilepsy; challenging behaviour.
Medical diagnosis: Renal failure.

Background

Donald lived in a residential group home with four other people with learning disabilities and attended a social services day centre on a full-time basis. A qualified LDN managed the home but did not actively practice as a nurse. The local bureaucracy of the joint association and health agreement dictates that he or she is unable to practice as a nurse within the home for liability and indemnity reasons. This had an enormous impact on the outcome of Donald's care. Other staff members were made up of healthcare assistants. Donald had quite a number of episodes of urinary infections, and was incontinent. Following a referral to his GP, urine and blood samples were forwarded for more detailed tests, which showed a large amount of protein and blood in his urine. These tests took place over a period of two months, after which a referral was made to the hospital renal unit where he underwent regular blood tests and urine analysis over a period of six months. He was given medication to ascertain any improvement. Following this period of treatment, the conclusion by the renal consultant was that he thought Donald would not be compliant with medical procedures and a diagnosis of terminal illness was made due to renal failure. The opinion was derived following evidence that Donald lacked tolerance to medical procedures (eg. needles, x-rays, medication) and was aggressive towards nursing staff during several admissions to hospital.

Donald's understanding of his illness

Donald had limited communication skills, but was aware of what was happening around him. It was felt by the staff that he had some understanding of his illness because his family became more involved and there were numerous and repeated visits to the doctors and hospital. He also stopped attending the day centre. Staff responses to him were also varied. Some staff at the day centre viewed his behaviour as 'attention-seeking' and subsequently difficult and challenging. They ignored his illness and did not recognise the reason for his behaviour. As a result, they were unable to continue to offer him a service.

Despite his illness, Donald presented as a fit and healthy young man, therefore giving a 'false' impression of his health. Staff felt very concerned and were unable to understand why Donald could not receive the same treatment and services available to the non-disabled population (eg. dialysis, kidney transplant or admission to palliative care services). The staff working with him in his home had diverse and different views of caring for him; some believed he should be told of his illness, others believed he should not. They were also unclear about his pain threshold and tolerance, and felt unable to assess his pain adequately due to the unavailability of appropriate pain-assessment tools from any of the services involved. They relied heavily on their knowledge of him, and their observational skills of his behaviour changes in determining his need for pain-relief medication. This resulted in an inconsistent pain-management regime.

Although there was excellent liaison and communication with primary and hospital healthcare teams, there were some difficulties in the day-to-day care for Donald. He was living in a two-storey home and there were concerns for both his and his staff's safety when using the stairs. The local housing association would not give permission for him to be cared for temporarily on the ground floor of the home (it would have contravened National Standard Commission regulations). Donald was therefore moved to another home nearby, and was cared for by strangers until his death a few weeks later. Staff felt saddened by this move, as they had cared for him for a number of years and were unable to be with him until the end of his life.

Agencies involved

The agencies involved in caring for Donald were numerous and included: the learning disability services who employed the staff of the home, the manager of which is a qualified LDN; the Primary Health Care Team, including the GP and District Nursing services; the local renal unit; and the Social Services Day Centre. The role of the LDN in this case was restricted due to local policy, meaning the LDN could not practise as a registered nurse. However, the training and experiences allowed her, as a manager of the unit, to:

1. Assess and recognise the individual holistic needs, which must be met by services.
2. Refer to other appropriate agencies for their specialist input, and organise emergency admission.
3. Identify the need for changes in local policy to provide care and service as the needs of the individual change from day to day.
4. Identify, liaise and communicate with all the services and agencies involved in this case.
5. Organise case reviews and update care plans.
6. Advise and support care staff and provide access to counselling and clinical supervision as necessary.
7. Supervise junior staff, to whom nursing functions were delegated. In this case, the manger of the home did not fully use the local Community Learning Disability Team (CLDN) to be the coordinator of this case, which would have given her the time for the other three people living in the home.
8. Facilitate access to appropriate counselling services, which should be available as an option to all the staff and other people living in the home.

Case Study Three

Name: Albert.
Age: 62.
Diagnosis: Learning disabilities.
Medical Diagnosis: Cancer of the spine.

Background

This elderly man lived with his sister after the death of his parents. He attended full time at the local Social Services Day Service. In addition to his basic reading and writing skills, his communication is very good and he is able to understand fully what is said to him. He has no sensory impairment. He is registered with the GP services in the area and, apart from the usual minor ailments, he never had cause to be seen by his doctor for any major medical problems until now.

Staff at the day centre recognised that something was 'just not right' and noticed that he took longer than usual to sit down or stand up. Walking was getting increasingly difficult for him, and he would stop several times to cover a 25m distance. Although Albert was not receiving any input from the local CLDT, an LDN (who did not cover the geographical area in which Albert lives, but visits the centre regularly) was approached for advice. After a period of observation and discussion with Albert, Albert's sister was advised to arrange an appointment with the GP, who requested investigative tests and screening. The day centre staff were advised to refer Albert to the CLDT responsible for that area.

After several weeks, an appointment was requested by the GP. At the appointment, Albert waited outside the consulting room while his sister was told that Albert had cancer and a referral would be made to the District Nursing service. No medication was prescribed for pain. Albert carried on attending the day centre as usual, and his sister awaited contact from the District Nurses. When this failed to materialise, the GP surgery was contacted and she was told over the phone that the doctor had made a mistake — it was the wrong diagnosis. It was therefore unnecessary to make a referral to the district nurses.

Another week passed and the sister was asked to attend the GP surgery with Albert. She, but not Albert, was told again that he had cancer. Albert noticed his sister's distress and started to ask questions about his more frequent visits to the doctors. No explanation was given. Two weeks later, the sister received a letter informing her that the tests show that Albert did not have cancer and that the pain he was experiencing was due to a kidney infection that eventually cleared up.

Although Albert was capable of understanding, at no time was information relating to his illness communicated to him personally. Every communication was conveyed through his sister without any offer of support and no apologies for the misunderstanding. This episode caused unnecessary anger and distress to the carer and could have been managed in a more honest, understanding and sensitive manner, with the individual's involvement.

Role of the LDN

In this case, a referral to the LDN would be appropriate and the nurse's role would involve offering:

1. Advice and support to Albert and his sister.
2. Advice, support and close liaison with the primary health care team (PHCT) and GP (involving the GP, district nursing services, screening services and hospital appointments) and clarifying and explaining diagnosis and information.
3. Providing education and advice to PHC services.
4. Acting as an advocate (or the person who refers to advocacy services) for Albert and his sister.

Figure 5.1: Services involved in providing holistic palliative care for the person with learning disabilities.

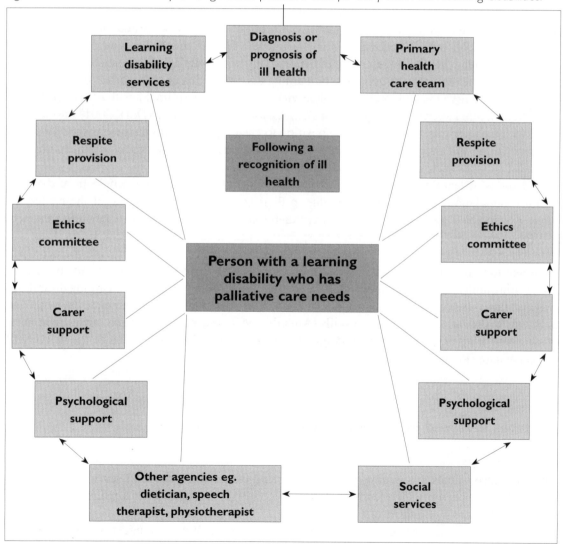

Although LDNs are not appropriately placed to make a diagnosis of cancer, their knowledge, skills and experience place them in a unique position to detect health changes and physical symptoms in individuals. The information they can provide to primary health care professionals can improve the care and attention given to people with learning disabilities. Keenan and McIntosh (2000) support this in their assertion that there is urgent need for closer working between palliative and learning-disability services.

Learning from the case studies

The three case studies have highlighted the important roles that LDNs have to ensure that people with learning disabilities who have palliative-care needs receive high-quality services. There is widespread recognition that people with learning disabilities receive poor-quality health care (DoH, 1998, 1999) and often symptoms are wrongly diagnosed and/or there are poor diagnoses of curative or non-curative illnesses (Tuffrey-Wijne, 1997; Hunt *et al*, 2001), resulting in inappropriate treatment. The Continuing the Commitment (1995) project not only described the knowledge and skills of the LDN, but also identified their key roles. This included the central role in health surveillance and promotion by working collaboratively with PHCT and specialist health services in meeting the health needs of people with learning disability: this can be a direct or indirect role in assessment, provision and evaluation of services to obtain the optimal health of the individual. The recent White Paper *Valuing People: a Strategy for the 21st Century* (DoH, 2001) provides the LDN with the opportunity to be in a key position to ensure people with learning disability access and receive the full range of health care, including their additional health requirements through specialist services such as palliative and terminal-care services.

People with learning disability are subject to physical illness (as are people from the non-disabled population), probably more so due to their learning disability. Some of these illnesses often go unnoticed and undiagnosed, and are therefore too far advanced to respond to treatment (Tuffrey-Wijne, 1997); others may not be responsive to curative treatment (Read, 1998). They will therefore require specialist health care (such as palliative care services) to provide the necessary treatment to maintain a good-quality and dignified lifestyle, whether they are cared for in their home or in another establishment. In addition to their illness, some people with learning disabilities will also face other challenges, such as social interaction, speech disorders, language development, problems with hearing and cognitive skills (Ambulu, 1997), and communication impairment (Kerr *et al*, 1996). Further, their individuality and uniqueness may affect and challenge the delivery of palliative care (Read, 1998).

Services involved in providing holistic palliative care

The three case studies in this chapter have illustrated the potential range of services that may be accessed by the person with a learning disability, following a diagnosis of a palliative condition. These services are highlighted in *Figure 5.1*.

Each of these services/agencies has a significant role within the context of palliative care.

Figure 5.2: Layers of support coordinated by the learning disability nurse (LDN).

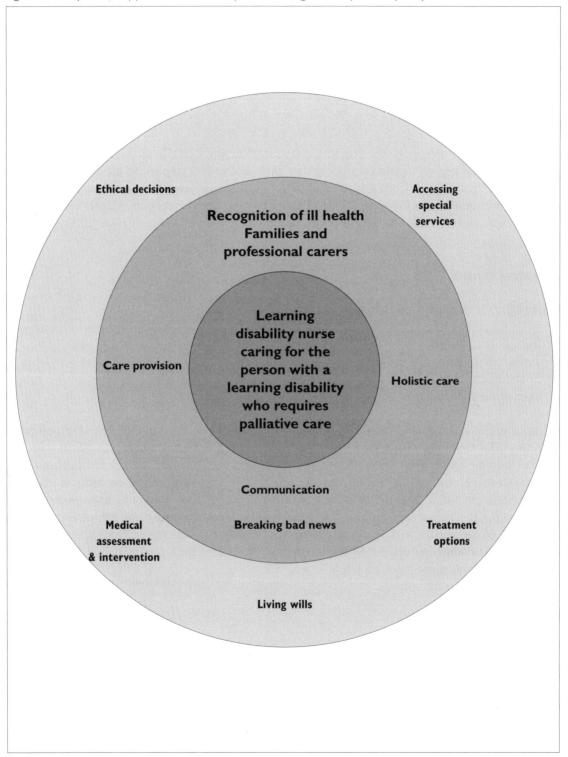

People with learning disabilities often have a number of professionals already working with them (Brown *et al*, 2003), and the diagnosis of palliative care needs and/or terminal illness will dictate the involvement of other professional groups. It is therefore important for the LDN to be an educator and coordinator within this context, so that each professional can clarify his or her individual role in providing a needs-led palliative care service for the person with learning disabilities.

Key roles for LDNs

The definition of nursing by the Royal College of Nursing (2003), as presented earlier, is a statement that all nurses should use to evaluate their tasks. This applies to all nurses, whatever their grade or speciality — from a nurse who works in palliative care who aims to maintain a good quality of life until death (Waters, 2003) to an LDN who should support people with learning disabilities to access health services designed around their individual needs (DoH, 2001).

Assessment of need

Jenkins (2002) identified four key roles for the LDN:

- assessment of need
- health surveillance and promotion
- enabling and empowering
- improving service quality.

Of these, assessment of need should be central to the LDN's role. Within the context of palliative care, the LDN should be able to use his or her experience and knowledge of various assessment tools to identify health need and/or design an assessment tool to meet individual needs, thereby enabling access to appropriate palliative care services. By empowering and enabling the person, the nurse will be able to help the individual make choices and give consent as appropriate.

Following the assessment process, the LDN will be able to identify and plan the palliative-care needs of the person with learning disabilities directly by working collaboratively with the client, carer and other appropriate professionals, and facilitating high-quality palliative care. Such 'layers' of care and support are shown in *Figure 5.2*.

Collaborative working

LDNs are in a pivotal position to work collaboratively with their health colleagues to meet the health needs of the people with learning disabilities. Hunt *et al* (2001) suggested that health professionals needed to share their skills and experience and establish networks that will signpost clients to user-friendly services. It is also crucial that information is shared between professionals prior to procedures and appointments, helping individuals cooperate and provide consent to treatment. This may involve pre-visits; meeting other professionals; using information and photographs; and getting used to unfamiliar environments. This will help to alleviate any anxiety, uncertainty and fears one may have when receiving new treatment in a strange environment.

Health promotion and education

It is vital for general health services to be prepared. *Signposts for Success* (DoH, 1998) suggests that LDNs should develop a facilitative and advisory role in helping other health staff to understand the needs of people with learning disability. Raising the awareness of health-care colleagues is part of the role of the LDN.

People with learning disabilities also need to be helped to understand their illness and the treatment required. The nurse has a vital role in educating and informing clients by way of health promotion (Kay, 1995; Mansell and Harris, 1998; Jenkins, 2002), using literature/information and visual aids, which can be adapted to suit individual needs. The provision of necessary information about illnesses and treatment leads to the individual's choice and consent to treatments, and the pictorial packages will be useful in clarifying and explaining procedures and treatment options (Hollins *et al*, 2000; DoH, 2003).

Figure 5.3: The diverse roles of the learning disability nurse (LDN).

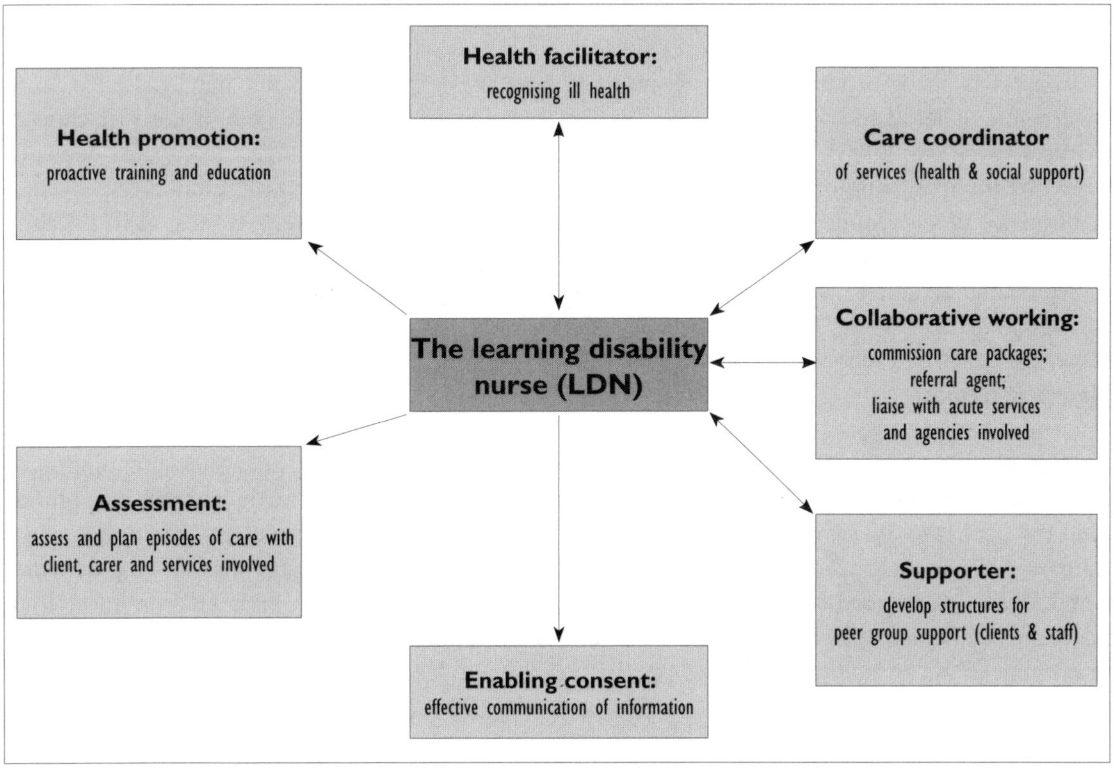

Enabling consent

Due to their varying level of communicative skills, people with learning disabilities may or may not be in a position to consent to their treatment (DoH, 2001, 2003). However, the person with a learning disability should be given clear and simple information using signs and visual aids where necessary to obtain his/her consent (DoH, 1995). The Nursing & Midwifery Council's *Code of Professional Conduct* (2002) advocates that voluntary consent must be received before treatment is given. If the person is not competent to give consent, treatment can be given in the person's best interest (DoH, 1999), but this must be the decision of the responsible medical professional. The LDN's skills and experience should enable them to work closely with palliative services in helping the individual to make choices and give — or withdraw — their consent.

Care coordinator

The LDN should ensure that the service the individual is receiving is well coordinated and effectively communicated (Sines, 1998) so that they benefit from the best health care that meets their palliative-care needs. This places the LDN in the position of 'manager of care', whereby services are commissioned and coordinated to meet the palliative care and holistic needs — medical, nursing, paramedical, day, respite, and support services — of the person concerned. Managers should be informed where there are deficits.

Supporter

Working with people with learning disabilities who are terminally ill and need palliative care treatment can leave the staff, clients and carers emotionally vulnerable and in need of support themselves (Read, 2003). The LDN is in an ideal position to acknowledge the support needs of everyone involved, and coordinate such needs. Within the caring profession, clinical supervision is one way of providing support (Fowler, 1996; Butterworth *et al*, 1998; Jones, 2001). While supporting clients, nurses and other professional carers must learn to recognise their own feelings of stress, and be able to access support, such as clinical supervision and personal counselling.

Health Facilitator

Valuing People (2001) identified the role of the health facilitator as ensuring the completion of health action plans — to facilitate, advocate and ensure that people with learning disabilities gain full access to primary and secondary health care. The difficulties this client group face when accessing generic services can be overcome if a health facilitator is appointed to support them. The LDN is well placed to take on this role. Their training, experiences and skills are more than adequate. Some agencies may already be aware of the difficulties faced by people and nominate or employ LDNs as facilitators between palliative care and learning-disability services. The person in this position can also serve as an advisor to primary health and palliative care services (DoH, 2001).

Another crucial role for the health facilitator is the development of an individual health action plan. If completed appropriately, it will inform the need for all appropriate service intervention for the person requiring the range of healthcare services to which they are entitled. This is a dynamic and evolving document that will change as the needs of the person change. Subsequently, the roles of the LDN in ensuring appropriate palliative care for people with learning disabilities may be numerous and diverse (see *Figure 5.3*).

Conclusion

The role of the LDN aims to support people with learning disabilities to live a full and independent lifestyle. Although diverse, the main objective is to commission, provide and support access to healthcare (including palliative care) to clients. Their training, knowledge, skills and wide range of experiences places them in an ideal position to bridge the gap between palliative care and learning disability services. This chapter has used case studies to reflect on the variety of skills used by the LDN from within a palliative care context. Services and agencies likely to be involved have been considered, and the key roles of the LDN identified and clarified.

People with learning disabilities have a range of complex, diverse needs and skills, which may present difficulties when they access palliative care services. These difficulties can be overcome if nurses are pro-active, seizing opportunities to work in collaboration with colleagues in primary and palliative services. They are resourceful and have the ability to develop new ways of working, not only improving the service to the individual but also improving their skills and experiences to meet the changing health needs of the people for whom they work.

It is important for LDNs to ensure that people with learning disabilities receive smooth and easy access to palliative care nursing services. The specialist training that they receive places them in a unique position, enabling them to work across professional boundaries and as intermediaries between service user and service.

With policy directives from *Valuing People* (DoH, 2001), the LDN needs to reflect on the wide diversity of their skill base. They need to adapt their knowledge and skills to improve their experience so that they can meet the challenge of the changes that face them. This will enable them to work in partnership with colleagues from all services. This can only lead to change and better service delivery of palliative care services for all people with learning disabilities.

References

Alaszewski A, Gates B, Motherby E, Manthorpe J, Ayer S (2001) Education programme for learning disability nursing: outcomes evaluation of the contribution of learning disability nurses within multi-professional, multi-agency teams. English National Board, London

Ambula S (1977) Communication. In: O'Hara J, Sperlinger A (eds) (1977) *Adults with Learning Disabilities: a Practical Approach for Health Professionals*. John Wiley & Sons, Chichester

Beacock C (1999) A bright future. *Learn Disabil Pract* **2**(3): 45–8

Boarder J (2002) The perceptions of experiences of community learning disability nurses of their roles and ways of working. *J Learn Disabil Health Soc Care* **6**(3): 281–96

Briggs A (1972) *DoH & Social Services: Report of the Committee on Nursing Project.* CMND 5115. HMSO, London

Brown H, Burns S, Flynn M (2003) Learning disability review: 'Please don't let it happen on my shift!" *Support Staff Caring People Learn Disabil Dying* **8**(2): 32–41

Butterworth T, Faugier J (1992) *Clinical Supervision and Mentorship in Nursing.* Chapman & Hall, London

DoH (1971) *Better Services for the Mentally Handicapped.* HMSO, London

DoH (1995) *Health of the Nation: a Strategy for People with Learning Disabilities.* HMSO, London

DoH (1996) *Mental Health (Patients in the Community) Act 1995.* Welsh Office

DoH (1998) *Signposts for Success in Commissioning and Providing Health Services for People with Learning Disabilities.* NHS Executive, London

DoH (1999) *Once a Day.* HMSO, London

DoH (1999) *Revised Mental Health Act 1983 Code of Practice.* HMSO, London

DoH (2000) *The National Cancer Plan: a Plan for Investment and Reform.* HMSO, London

DoH (2001) *Valuing People: a Strategy for the 21ˢᵗ Century.* HMSO, London

DoH (2001) *Reference Guide to Consent for Examination or Treatment.* HMSO, London

DoH (2003) Seeking Consent: working with people with learning disabilities. HMSO, London

Fowler J (1996) The organisation of clinical supervision within nursing professions: a review of the literature. *J Adv Nurs* **23**: 471–8

Hollins S, Downer J (2000) *Keeping Healthy 'Down Below'.* St George's Medical School, London

Howells G (1997) A general perspective. In: O'Hara J, Sperlinger A (eds) (1977) *Adults with Learning Disabilities: a Practical Approach for Health Professionals.* John Wiley & Sons, Chichester

Hunt C, Wakefield S, Hunt G (2001) Community nurses in learning disability: a case study of the use of evidence-based screening tools to identify and meet the health needs of people with learning disabilities. *Int J Learn Disabil* **5**(1): 78–80

Jancar J (1988) Consequences of a longer life for the mentally handicapped. *Geriatr Med* **5**: 81–7

Jancar MP, Jancar J (1977) Cancer and mental retardation. *Bristol Med Chir J* **92**: 3–7

Jay P (1979) *Report of the Committee of the Inquiry into Mental Handicap Nursing.* HMSO, London

Jenkins R (2002) Enhancing quality of life for people with learning disabilities. *Learn Disabil Pract* **5**(9): 102–5

Jones A (2001) Possible influences on clinical supervision. *Nurs Stand* **16**(1): 38–42

Kay B, Rose S, Turnbull J (1995) *Continuing the Commitment: the Report of the Learning*

Disability Nursing Project. DoH, London

Keenan P, McIntosh P (2000) Learning disabilities and palliative care. *Palliat Care Today* **14**: 11–14

Kerr M, Fraser W, Felce D (1996) Primary health care for people with a learning disability. *Br J Learn Disabil* **24**: 2–8

Lott I, McCoy E (1992) *Down Syndrome: Advances in Medical Care*. Wiley Publishing, New York

Mencap (1998) *The NHS — Health for All? People with Learning Disability and Healthcare*. Mencap National Centre, London

Nursing & Midwifery Council (2002) *Code of Professional Conduct*. NMC, London

Read S (1998) The palliative care needs of people with learning disabilities. *J Palliat Nurs* **4**(5): 246–51

Read S (2003) Bereavement and loss. In: Markwick A, Parrish A (2003) *Learning Disability: Themes and Perspectives*. Butterworth-Heinemann, UK

Royal College of Nursing (2003) *Defining Nursing*. RCN, London

Sines D (1998) Nursing intervention. In: Fraser W, Sines D, Kerr M (eds) (1998) *The Care of People with Intellectual Disabilities*. Butterworth-Heinnemann, UK

Sperlinger A, O'Hara J (eds) (1997) *Adults with Learning Disabilities: a Practical Approach for Health Professionals*. John Wiley & Sons, Chichester

Stanley R (1998) Primary health care provision for people with learning disability: a survey of general practitioners. *J Learn Disabil Health Soc Care* **2**(1): 23–30

Tuffrey-Wijne I (1997) Palliative care and learning disabilities. *Nurs Times* **93**(31): 50–1

Waters A (2003) What is nursing? *Nurs Stand* **17**(31): 20–2

CHAPTER 6

Ethical decision-making

Karen Ryan, Regina McQuillan

A man without ethics is a wild beast loosed upon this world.
   Albert Camus (1913–1960), novelist, essayist and playwright

Ethics is the study of morality: it asks questions about how we ought to act, and how we should live. Answers to these questions have been debated since the time of Aristotle, yet a range of possible responses still exists to any specific ethical issue. This is because ethical decision-making involves an expression of a person's values, and a person's value system depends largely on his or her own philosophical, theological and cultural perspectives and experiences. Values are those things that are important to, or valued by, someone. Values determine whether a person feels that they are doing right or wrong; whether an action is worthwhile or desirable. Members of a postmodern society can have many diverse values and this can lead to difficulties for the individual, and for society as a whole, who have to weigh and prioritise competing values in order to make decisions on ethical issues.

This chapter will provide an introduction to some of the central ethical issues encountered by health and social care workers when caring for a person with learning disability towards the end of life. Although the issues are largely similar to those that are encountered in the palliative care of the general population, the context in which they arise is significantly different, and this has important implications for their management. Social and health services traditionally operate with very different types of skill-mix and value-base. The social model of disability understands disability as the loss or limitation of opportunities to take part in the normal life of the community on an equal level with others due to physical and social barriers (DPI, 1982). The medical model of disability focuses on the person with impairment, and does not consider the disabling structures of society; it considers disability to be the result of a physical condition, and as such interventions are directed at rehabilitation or 'cure'.

A healthcare provider's personal values can influence his or her attitudes towards the type of care that he or she feels a person with learning disability should receive. Attitudinal barriers can obstruct access to care (Aunos and Feldman, 2002; NHS Cancer Screening Programme, 2000) and it has been shown that people with learning disabilities and advanced disease are not always offered the same treatment options as the general population at the end of life (Northfield and Turnbull, 2001). Although people with learning disabilities more commonly have difficulty accessing general healthcare services due to the attitudes of general healthcare staff, attitudes of learning-disability staff can also affect care. The Growing Older with Learning Disabilities Programme found evidence that some learning-disability services did not consider hospice care, even when it was considered appropriate, because of previous poor experiences of the acute care system (Brown *et al*, 2002). Important ethical issues are raised by these examples of the difficulties faced by people with learning disabilities in gaining access to services generally, and palliative care in particular.

The few case studies published on palliative-care provision and people with learning disability have pointed to additional ethical issues (Tuffrey-Wijne, 1997, 2002). Issues of communication, truth-telling and consent have been shown to pose challenges to both learning disability and healthcare professionals. The rapid advances that have taken place in health care have further complicated the situation. Researchers have pushed the boundaries of medicine so far that it is now possible to carry out procedures that were not even thought of a few decades ago, resulting in a widening gap between the perspectives of healthcare professionals and the public.

Within the scope of this chapter, it was not possible to consider comprehensively all the ethical issues encountered at the end of life, and inevitably we had to sacrifice discussion of certain topics. We did not include a discussion on euthanasia and physician-assisted suicide because our focus was on giving the reader an awareness of common ethical issues that arise when providing palliative care to a person with learning disability. We do acknowledge, however, the central importance of this subject to society, and we recognise that debate on the subjects of euthanasia and physician-assisted suicide has achieved particular intensity in recent years (as evidenced by the proposed *Assisted Dying for the Terminally Ill Bill* currently being debated in the UK parliament). The subject has particular relevance for people with learning disability because of the centrality to the debate of the concepts of autonomy and value of life.

Approaches to ethical decision-making

Approaches to ethical decision-making are rational or non-rational. The term 'non-rational' does not mean that the decision-making process is irrational; rather, it simply means the approach does not use a process of reasoning that involves considering both the arguments for and against a particular decision. Non-rational approaches include obedience; following the example of a role model; or operating according to habit or instinct. Such approaches are often used in day-to-day life, but they have shortcomings: they are largely subjective in nature and decisions can vary significantly from person to person; also, in the event of ethical conflict, the approaches provide little common ground for discussion between concerned parties.

Ethics primarily concerns itself with rational approaches to decision-making, and the main traditions are outlined in *Panel 6.1*. Of the different approaches, the four-principle system has become increasingly influential in healthcare ethics in recent years (Beauchamp and Childress, 2001). Beauchamp and Childress argue that members of society share a common morality, and from this they deduce principles that should be used in decision-making in medical ethics. The four principles are *prima facie* duties, which means that they are considered always to be in effect. There is no intrinsic hierarchy to the principles; they are all of equal weight, all other things being

---

Panel 6.1: **Common ethical frameworks**

- **Deontology**
  Deontological approaches have the concept of 'duty' as the basis for the decision-making process. Duties can be understood as clear obligations that guide ethical action, although there are different theories as to what constitutes a duty. Some examples are the duty of honesty or the duty to treat people as an end and never as a means to an end. However, problems can arise in situations where a person must choose between two conflicting duties. There can also be difficulties when harm is caused in the process of acting according to duty.

- **Consequentialism**
  This approach is often contrasted with that of deontology because consequentialists base their ethical decision-making on an analysis of the likely consequences of actions. The right action is said to be the one that produces the best outcome. Individuals may disagree as to what constitutes the 'best outcome', however, and may challenge whether the end always justifies the means.

- **Virtue ethics**
  Virtue ethicists place less emphasis on following defined rules of conduct and instead stress the importance of developing good habits of character. Virtues are attitudes or character traits that enable us to achieve the full potential of our humanity, such as honesty, compassion and courage. It can be argued, in spite of this, that even virtuous people can make the wrong decisions.

- **Principlism**
  This approach uses ethical principles as the basis of making decisions. The four principles that are commonly invoked as guides are *respect for autonomy, beneficence, non-maleficence* and *justice*. Ethicists apply the principles to particular cases, taking into account both rules and consequences, in the process of deciding what is the right thing to do. Situations can arise, nevertheless, when the principles conflict and an ethicist may then have to prioritise one principle over another. It should also be remembered that these four principles have emerged from the context of Western liberal culture and are not necessarily universal. *Beneficence* means doing good; *non-maleficence* means doing no harm; *justice* refers to treating like cases alike, and distributing benefits and burdens fairly; *respect for autonomy* means respecting people's decisions.

---

equal. Ethical dilemmas are said to arise when two or more of the principles come into conflict and a person's course of action is then determined by weighing and balancing all competing *prima facie* duties in any particular case.

How to choose an approach to ethical decision-making

People generally choose their favoured approach to decision-making on the basis of their own beliefs and values, and a certain approach will often intuitively 'feel right' to that person. As individuals gain a more sophisticated understanding of ethics, they will choose an approach on the basis of a considered judgement. Members of a particular group or profession often share common values and therefore specific groups may show preferences for specific approaches to decision-making. It is thus very important that a person has a general understanding of all approaches to ethical decision-making so that he or she can understand the reasoning behind other peoples' decisions.

Each approach helps us to make an ethical decision, but there are still problems to be resolved. The first is that people might not always agree on how to apply a specific approach to particular circumstances. The case of a person with a severe learning disability who has advanced lung cancer and who has an extreme phobia to needles demonstrates this problem. The oncologist tells the carers that chemotherapy is likely only to prolong the person's survival by a matter of weeks, but that it may help to control the symptoms of the disease. In such cases, it is not always clear what constitutes 'benefit' and what constitutes 'harm'.

The second problem is more fundamental, and difficult to resolve. It arises when the approaches do not answer the question of 'what is the ethical decision?' in the same way. Common responses in such a circumstance are:

- To reflect further on the ethical issue, and to try to determine which solution is the strongest — ie. is focused on values and stakeholders of most importance to the case.
- To develop a creative alternative solution that satisfies all ethical principles.
- To act in a manner that incorporates all possible solutions, if this is possible.
- To consult an independent third party, such as an ethics committee.

Making decisions that involve people with learning disabilities: evidence from the literature

Most of the research that has been carried out on the subject of decision-making by, and for, people with learning disabilities has focused on general healthcare issues, rather than on end-of-life concerns. We know that many adults with learning disabilities are not involved in decisions about their own general healthcare (Keywood *et al*, 1999). We also know that the decisions that carers make on behalf of people with learning disabilities are made without proper attention to ethical issues — for example, making decisions on the basis of an assumption of incompetence or failing to consider the best interests standard (Keywood *et al*, 1999; Holloway, 2004). Recognising that people become increasingly vulnerable towards the end of life, it would seem reasonable to extrapolate from this data that the autonomy of people with learning disabilities may be further compromised at this time. This underlines the importance of the need for health and social care workers to have an explicit commitment to addressing these issues in practice.

Management of ethical issues in clinical practice

Ethical issues are not all equally challenging. Some may be relatively easy to answer, particularly if there is already a well-developed consensus on the right way to act in the situation; however, more complex issues are common. Ethical dilemmas occur in situations where all options have some value, and when making the decision means that one set of values has been chosen at the expense of others. In more complicated cases, it may be helpful to follow the steps of an ethical decision-making model to assess which of the ethical principles may be in conflict. One such model involves the following steps (Williams JR, 2005):

1. Determine whether the issue at hand is an ethical one.
2. Consult authoritative sources, such as professional codes of ethics, published policies and respected colleagues to see how similar issues are generally dealt with.
3. Consider alternative solutions in light of the principles and values that they uphold and their likely consequences.
4. Discuss your proposed solution with those whom it will affect.
5. Make your decision and act on it with sensitivity to others affected.
6. Evaluate your decision and be prepared to act differently in the future.

Reference is made to the use of codes of ethics because they are an important resource for healthcare professionals. No two codes of ethics are identical as they reflect the values of the professional group. They are not supposed to define everything that constitutes ethical behaviour, but they are a starting point for the definition of minimal behaviour acceptable to the group. As such, violations of codes of conduct are usually taken very seriously, and any member who breaches his or her professional code of conduct should be prepared to face possible disciplinary action.

Ethical decisions about end-of-life care have the potential to impact profoundly on all those involved in, and affected by, the decision-making process (Doka K, 2005). They may complicate the grief of those who live on by creating dissent between carers, or by increasing ambivalence over the circumstances of death; but they may also facilitate the grief process when handled well. Communication and reflective practice are central to this process and their importance is recognised in steps 4 to 6 of the model.

Management of ethical conflict and clinical practice

Disagreements about healthcare decisions can arise between or among any of the following: the person receiving care; family members; care providers; and administrators of healthcare authorities. Various models have been proposed, but the following is adapted from the Joint Statement on Preventing and Resolving Ethical Conflicts Involving Health Care Providers and Persons Receiving Care, which was developed by the Boards of Directors of the Canadian Healthcare Association, the Canadian Medical Association, the Canadian Nurses Association and the Catholic Health Association of Canada (1999).

The first step towards resolving conflict involves gathering the involved parties together in order to establish communication. It may be necessary or advisable to have a person who is not involved in the conflict to mediate the dispute, and such a person should have experience of conflict-resolution. Communication should initially focus on identification of points of agreement and disagreement. The roles and responsibilities of each participant should also be established.

Next, all options should be identified and a time schedule determined for resolving the conflict. If, after reasonable effort, agreement or compromise cannot be reached through dialogue, the decision of the person with the right or responsibility for making the decision should be accepted. If it is unclear or disputed who has the right or responsibility to make the decision, then adjudication to an ethics committee or legal body should be sought. Once the process is completed, the process, the decision reached and its implementation should be reviewed and evaluated.

Confidentiality and informed consent (*Case Study 1*)

Case Study 1: John

John is a thirty-four year-old man with Down syndrome and a mild learning disability. His parents died some years ago. He has one brother who is forty-five years old. John lives alone and has a full-time job in supported employment. He recently noted a swelling of his testicles and went to his GP, Dr Brown. John is aware of recent public-health campaigns that have focused on men's health, and is very worried that the swelling might be due to cancer. Dr Brown examines John and is also concerned that testicular cancer is causing the swelling. He immediately arranges for further tests at the local hospital, but tells John not to worry because 'it's nothing serious'. After John has left the surgery, Dr Brown rings John's brother to inform him of his concerns and to let him know about the planned investigations.

Case Study 1 focuses on the ethical issues of informed consent and confidentiality. Both issues are underpinned by the principle of respect for autonomy, and both are protected in law. Autonomy may be understood as the right of the individual to self-determination, and this is acknowledged in clinical practice by the process of obtaining informed consent. Respect for the privacy of an individual is also central to respect for autonomy, and this is acknowledged by the practice of confidentiality.

In the example above, Dr Brown breached confidentiality by discussing John's case with his brother without first seeking permission to do so. Confidential information should only be disclosed in exceptional circumstances, such as when it is judged to be in the patient's best interests or when in is necessary to do so to protect society. Rarely, it may be necessary to break confidentiality when there is a legal obligation to do so (General Medical Council [GMC], 2000). Confidentiality is central to trust between healthcare professionals and their patients. Unless patients are certain that confidentiality will be respected, they may be reluctant to give healthcare professionals the information that they need to provide good care.

Both learning-disability and palliative-care practitioners work in the multidisciplinary setting, and it is usual practice to share information about the patient within the team in order to provide good care to that patent. Patients should therefore be made aware that, unless they object, information will be shared. The reasons for this should be explained to them. Family members are also central to the care of a person with learning disabilities and occupy a valued place in that person's social world. They have an understandable desire to receive healthcare information about their relative, but it is important to respect confidentiality by obtaining consent for disclosure from the person with learning disabilities first. The right to confidentiality can be overridden in situations when it is deemed to be in the learning-disabled's best interests — for example, in order to protect the person's safety or to prevent abuse.

In *Case Study 1*, Dr Brown gave John misleading information about the investigations and thereby failed to get informed consent. Consent may be described as the 'autonomous authorisation of a medical intervention... by individual patients' (Beauchamp and Faden, 1995). It allows individuals the equal right to accept or refuse the proposed intervention. It has three components: disclosure, capacity and voluntariness. 'Disclosure' refers to the provision of sufficient information to a person about his or her condition and treatment options. 'Capacity' refers to a person's ability to understand information relevant to a treatment decision, and to appreciate the likely consequences of a decision or lack of decision. 'Voluntariness' refers to the patient's right to come to a decision freely, without undue influence.

Dr Brown might have been motivated by a belief that John was incapable of making decisions for himself when he organised the investigations, but he did not inform John of their purpose. This approach to decision-making is referred to as the 'status' approach, and was commonly used in the past when those with a low IQ, such as people with learning disability, were automatically considered to be incompetent. In recent years, this approach has been rejected for being 'out of tune with the policy aim of enabling and encouraging people to take for themselves any decision which they have capacity to take' (Law Commission of England and Wales Mental Incapacity, 1995) and the 'functional' approach to capacity is used instead. This approach recognises that capacity arises in a specific context, such as capacity to make a will or the ability to consent to medical treatment. It also views capacity as being time-specific, as well as issue-specific, and allows for fluctuating states of capacity. The time-specific aspect of capacity is of particular importance in the palliative-care setting, because delirium commonly occurs towards the end of life. The cognitive impairment associated with this condition characteristically varies in severity, allowing for the possibility that a person's level of capacity may also change with time.

In law, adults are presumed to possess capacity unless it is demonstrated otherwise. However, capacity is a complex concept and can be difficult to assess. The more serious the possible consequences of a decision, the greater the corresponding level of capacity required to make the decision. Considerable work has therefore been put into developing clinical tools to assess capacity in order to consent to healthcare procedures. The Department of Health (DoH) and the Lord Chancellor's Department have also drafted guidance, and point to factors that might negatively impact on assessment of capacity, such as inadequate time for consultation with a patient or failure to use aides to communication (Lord Chancellor's Department, 2003a-f). The Mental Capacity Act (2005) will provide additional guidance in a code of practice that will accompany the legislation when it comes into force (Department for Constitutional Affairs Mental Capacity Bill: Draft Code of Practice, 2004).

Incapacity and the Best Interests Standard (*Case Study 2*)

> ### *Case Study 2: Sarah*
>
> Sarah is a twenty-eight year-old lady with cerebral palsy and a profound learning disability. She has spastic quadriplegia and has developed a large pressure sore, which has failed to respond to treatment and is causing Sarah a great deal of pain. Sarah has been hospitalised on numerous occasions over the course of her lifetime and now appears to become distressed whenever she stays there. She becomes particularly distressed when she receives injections or when blood is taken from her. The consultant who reviews Sarah in the out-patient clinic recommends that Sarah be admitted to hospital and that a skin graft be performed in order to heal the pressure sore. Her parents are concerned that this would actually cause Sarah more harm than good and they refuse to go along with the plan.

When a person is judged to be incompetent to make a specific decision, then it is necessary for someone else to make the decision on behalf of the incompetent person. The laws that govern this process vary from country to country, and are presently undergoing significant review in England and Wales because of the introduction of the Mental Capacity Act (2005). This act received Royal Assent in April 2005 and will be implemented in 2007. It will provide a framework for acting and making decisions on behalf of individuals who lack mental capacity to make these decisions.

At present, in England and Wales, decisions about the medical care of the incompetent patient are the responsibility of his or her medical team. The decision-making process is based on the best-interests standard — that is, it is the patient's best interests that are relevant, not those of the decision-maker or anyone else. The views of people who knew the incapacitated person's feelings and values may be taken into account; however, priority is given to what is objectively the best course of action for the person lacking capacity. In *Case Study 2*, therefore, the consultant needs to determine what is in Sarah's best interests by exploring the ethical dimensions of the case further.

The Adults with Incapacity (Scotland) Act (2000) regulates intervention in the affairs of adults who have impaired capacity in Scotland. The guiding principles of the Act are that interventions must benefit the adult and take account of his or her wishes, so far as these can be ascertained. Interventions must also take account of the views of relevant others as far as it is reasonable and practical to do so, and restrict the adult's freedom as little as possible while still achieving the desired benefit.

A welfare attorney, a person authorised under an intervention order or a welfare guardian with powers relating to the medical treatment in question may give consent to medical treatment on behalf of an incapacitated adult. Doctors may provide essential medical treatment in an emergency, unless there is evidence of a valid advance refusal of a particular treatment. Other than in an emergency, or where there is a proxy decision-maker, a certificate of incapacity must be issued to provide care or treatment. Certain procedures must be followed if there is disagreement about an adult's treatment; these procedures may involve obtaining a second medical opinion. An application may be made to court if the disagreement is not resolved.

The Mental Capacity Act (2005)

The Mental Capacity Act (2005) will significantly change current law and practice in relation to the care and treatment of adults who lack capacity. It will cover decision-making for adults who lose capacity at some point in their lives, and also for adults whose incapacitating condition has been present since birth. The need for change in legislation became apparent following reports that formed the basis for the Green Paper *Who Decides? — Making Decisions on Behalf of Mentally Incapacitated Adults* (1997). Indeed, the then Lord Chancellor stated in his announcement to the UK's House of Lords:

> *The law is confusing and fragmented. Many carers in particular are expected to make decisions on behalf of incapacitated adults without a clear idea as to the legal authority for those decisions.*

The key principles that apply to all decisions and actions taken under the Act are:

- A person must be assumed to have capacity unless it is established that he lacks capacity.
- A person is not to be treated as unable to make a decision unless all practicable steps to help him to do so have been taken without success.
- A person is not to be treated as unable to make a decision merely because he makes an unwise decision.
- An act done, or decision made, under this Act for or on behalf of a person who lacks capacity must be done, or made, in his best interests.
- Before the act is done, or the decision is made, regard must be had to whether the purpose for which it is needed can be as effectively achieved in a way that is less restrictive of the person's rights and freedom of action.

The first part of the Act defines 'persons who lack capacity'. It contains a set of key principles and sets out a checklist to be used in ascertaining a person's best interests. It establishes a new statutory scheme for 'lasting' powers of attorney, and allows attorneys to have the authority to make healthcare decisions. The Act describes the jurisdiction of the new Court of Protection to make declarations and orders and to appoint substitute decision-makers ('deputies'), where a person lacks capacity. It also establishes a new statutory official, the Public Guardian, to support the work of the court.

Rules are set out about advance decisions to refuse medical treatment and new safeguards are established to protect adults without capacity who participate in research. The Act also establishes a system for providing independent mental capacity advocates for particularly vulnerable people. The Act introduces a new criminal offence of ill treatment or neglect of a person who lacks capacity, and deals with liability for actions in connection with the care or treatment of an incapacitated adult.

Many of the provisions in the Act are based on principles that have already been established in law through decisions made by courts in individual cases. The Act aims to clarify several legal uncertainties and to reform and update the current law where decisions need to be made on behalf of others. The Act will be accompanied by a Code of Practice that will provide guidance to all those working with and/or caring for adults who lack capacity and will describe their responsibilities.

Anticipatory decision-making and substituted judgement

Advance directives are a form of anticipatory decision-making. They allow adults with capacity to make a decision in advance to refuse specified treatments in the event of losing capacity in the future. Neither competent nor incompetent patients have the right to demand specific forms of treatment, so advance directives cannot instruct doctors to give treatments that they consider clinically unnecessary, futile or inappropriate. Although requests and preferences for treatment do not carry legal weight, good practice dictates that they should at least be listened to and considered. Doctors clearly cannot be instructed to give unlawful interventions, such as euthanasia.

The British Medical Association (BMA) recognises possible advantages of advance directives, but points to some possible disadvantages also (BMA, 1995). Advance decisions cannot encompass unforeseen possibilities and options, and medical practice is always evolving. There is always the possibility of a mistaken diagnosis, and views may change as to what constitutes a tolerable existence. Nevertheless, advance directives are one way of seeking to promote patient choice.

As already stated, a person may be nominated to act as surrogate decision-maker under the new form of power of attorney. The Attorney should use the best interests principle to determine what decision to make on behalf of the incapacitated person. The Act sets out some statutory guidance on how a person's best interests should be determined in the form of a checklist of common factors that should always be taken into account. This method of decision-making is in contrast to that used in other countries where decision-makers base their decisions on the following hierarchy of evidence:

- Explicit directive — ie. the instructions expressed by the patient when possessing capacity
- Substituted judgment — ie. inferences about what the patient would likely want in this situation, based on what is known about his prior behaviour and decision-making
- Best interest — ie. what the surrogate and healthcare team believe is best for the patient.

Truth-telling and communication (*Case Study 3*)

Problems around truth-telling are not unique to people with learning disabilities because it is a natural instinct for family members to try to protect their relative from knowledge of the incurable nature of an illness. Carers of an individual with learning disability are often particularly concerned about the effects such information would have on the coping strategy of an individual, and often use such arguments as 'he won't understand' or 'the truth is too upsetting'.

There are a number of important arguments in favour of truth-telling (Randall and Downie, 1999). The first is that society holds a fundamental belief in the value of truth and, as such, it

> **Case Study 3: Peter**
>
> Peter is nineteen years-old and has congenital myotonic dystrophy and a moderate learning disability. He has respiratory difficulties due to muscle atrophy, and has suffered recurrent aspiration pneumonias. His family are aware that his general condition has been steadily deteriorating in recent months and that the team caring for Peter feel that his prognosis is likely to be measured in weeks. His grandfather, to whom he was very close, died two years ago.
>
> Peter has already remarked to his family that he feels unwell and that he isn't able to do the things that he used to be able to manage. He appears low in mood and is tearful at times. He has started asking his family whether he will get better and he talks about his grandfather more often than previously. Peter's family try to reassure him that he will get better, but it doesn't seem to improve his spirits.

has intrinsic worth. Second, truth forms the basis of the trust that is essential to the patient-carer relationship. Third, people need the information to allow them to make authentic choices about treatment and life issues. It is worth considering that people with learning disabilities often already lack control and choices in their lives, and the maintenance of a 'conspiracy of silence' can result in further loss of autonomy.

The possibility that truth-telling may actually cause harm to the individual acts as a counter-balance to these arguments. There may indeed be individual circumstances that make the risk of harm to the individual likely, such as a specific and relevant psychiatric history. In such cases, careful consideration of the ethical issues may find that the best interests of the patient are served by withholding information. In the general population, there has been little hard evidence found to suggest that truth-telling is harmful. In fact, in one series of 101 patients with inoperable tumours, those who were not told about their condition had the highest rates of drug use, anxiety and depression (Gerle *et al*, 1960). Unfortunately, there are not any similar studies that examine its effects in people with learning disability.

If one agrees with the principle of truth-telling, then the next question that arises is: how much of the truth is it appropriate to tell? (Ellis and Tattershall, 1999). Current practice in Western society is that the patient is told 'as much of the truth as they want to know'. This position allows individuals to make their own choices as to the amount of information that they receive, and has the theoretical benefit of allowing them to receive information at a rate that they can cope with. However, there are potential limitations to this approach when considering people with learning disability — the person may not understand the need to ask questions in order to get the information required, or may not understand the subtlety of the 'warning shot'. There is clearly a need to adapt traditional models of breaking bad news to the individual needs of people with learning disabilities (McEnhill, 2004) and to use different communication aides to support this process.

Withdrawing and withholding conventional treatment (*Case Study 4*)

Case Study 4: Mary

Mary is a fifty-six year-old lady with Down syndrome and Alzheimer's disease who lives in a specialist unit providing care for people with dementia. She was diagnosed with dementia five years ago, but in recent months her overall condition has deteriorated significantly. The possibility of placing a feeding tube was discussed when Mary's condition began to worsen, and was decided against. Her communication is now minimal and she is dependent on others for activities of daily living (ADL). She has suffered recurrent aspiration pneumonias, and has received three courses of antibiotics in recent weeks. Her family wish to meet with the team caring for Mary in order to plan her ongoing care. They wish to consider what measures are appropriate to treat her next infection, and although they agreed with the decision not to place a feeding tube, they do now have some concerns about maintaining her fluid intake.

The primary goal of medical treatment is to benefit patients by restoring or maintaining their health as far as possible. In some circumstances, it is not possible to do this, and the justification for intervention is called into question. It can be argued that medicine's goal is not to prolong life at all costs, and that consideration should also be given to a person's quality of life. This is an expression of the principle of proportionality, which holds that life-prolonging treatments are contraindicated when they cause more suffering than benefit.

Although emotionally it may be easier to withhold treatment than to withdraw it, there are no legal differences between the two actions. It is clear that treatment should never be withheld when there is a possibility that it will benefit the patient, simply because withholding is considered to be easier than withdrawing treatment. It is important to note that we are not speaking of the practices of euthanasia or physician-assisted suicide when we refer to the withholding or withdrawal of life-prolonging treatment.

Decisions about withdrawing or withholding treatment can be difficult to make when there is disagreement between stakeholders about the treatment's relative burdens and benefits. Good communication is central to working through this debate. It is also advisable to look towards the literature for any evidence-based guidelines that might have previously been published in the area, and that might provide direction (BMA, 2001; GMC, 2002). When reasonable doubt exists about the potential for benefit, then a possible solution is to provide treatment for a trial period with a clear timeframe set in advance for its review.

Withdrawing and withholding treatment: artificial hydration and nutrition

The issue of whether it is ethically permissible to withdraw artificial nutrition and hydration is a contentious one. The UK House of Lords confirmed that these interventions are classed as medical treatment in the case of Tony Bland (Airedale NHS Trust *vs* Bland, 1993). However, many people still believe that the withdrawal of artificial nutrition or hydration is fundamentally different to the withdrawal of other medical treatments. This is due to a belief that nutrition and hydration, even when administered artificially, are basic human rights and therefore should not be regarded as medical interventions. Due to the sensitive and complex nature of such decisions, the English courts decided that a court declaration should be sought in all cases where it is proposed to withdraw artificial nutrition and hydration. However, this guidance only refers to patients in a persistent vegetative state (PVS). The position for other patients in similar circumstances, such as patients with dementia, is unclear. Healthcare teams should be aware that withdrawal of artificial nutrition and hydration from these patients could be challenged in the courts. It is recommended that the healthcare team, those close to the patient and a second or expert opinion should be sought before withdrawing treatment in such circumstances (GMC, 2002).

Both the BMA and the National Council for Hospice and Specialist Palliative Care Services (Joint Working Party between the National Council for Hospice and Specialist Palliative Care Services and the Ethics Committee of the Association for Palliative Medicine of Great Britain and Ireland, 2002) recognise that continuing artificial nutrition and hydration may not it be in the best interests of the imminently dying patient. In such circumstances, intervention should be withdrawn and the National Council for Hospice and Specialist Palliative Care Services provides background information on the subject in order to assist in the decision-making process. In the document *Ethical Decision Making in Palliative Care: Artificial Hydration for People who are Terminally Ill*, they state that:

- A blanket policy of artificial hydration, or of no artificial hydration, is ethically indefensible.
- Towards death, a person's desire for food and drink lessens. Study evidence is limited but suggests that artificial hydration in imminently dying patients influences neither survival nor symptom control. As such, it may constitute an unnecessary intrusion.
- Thirst or dry mouth in people who are terminally ill may frequently be caused by medication. In such circumstances, artificial hydration is unlikely to alleviate the symptom. Good mouth care and reassessment of medication become the most appropriate interventions.
- Appropriate palliative care will involve consideration of the option of artificial hydration, where dehydration results from a potentially correctable cause (eg. recurrent vomiting or hypercalcaemia).
- It is a responsibility of the clinical team to make assessments concerning the relevance of hydration to the experience of individual patients. Its appropriateness should be judged on a day-to-day basis, weighing up the potential harms and benefits.
- Relatives at the bedside of dying patients frequently express concern about lack of fluid or nutrient intake. Healthcare professionals should try to address those anxieties, but should always act in the best interests of their patients.

In *Case Study 4*, Mary's clinical condition is deteriorating rapidly and it is appropriate to reconsider goals of care. This might be done in the following manner. The first thing to do is to establish the facts of the situation. Mary is clearly weakening and it is important to find out the opinion of her medical team on what is the likely course of her illness and what is her possible prognosis. Assuming that they tell her family that she is in the terminal phase of her illness and that she is very likely to develop another aspiration pneumonia in the coming days or short weeks, then the next question is: what benefit would further antibiotics have for her? In reply, the team say that Mary has only shown a partial response to her last course of antibiotic therapy, and that her overall condition has continued to deteriorate, despite their use. They do not feel that further courses of antibiotics would have better effect and tell her family that, at best, antibiotics may provide some relief from the symptoms of pneumonia only. In addition, they say that there are alternative medications that can provide symptomatic relief, but that can be administered in a less invasive way. Mary's family and the team consider this information. They decide that it would be in Mary's best interests if the focus of care were now entirely palliative in intent, and if antibiotic therapy were withheld in the event of a further pneumonia, while at the same time all measures to maintain her comfort were pursued.

Mary's family and the team now consider issues of nutrition and hydration. Her family are made aware that in view of Mary's repeated aspiration of oropharyngeal secretions, and rapidly deteriorating condition, artificial nutrition would have no impact on survival. Mary has shown little interest in food for many weeks now, and her family are reassured that she is not suffering because of this. When considering the issue of hydration, however, her family state that on occasion they feel that she is looking for something to drink. In view of this and the fact that Mary is not imminently dying but could live some short weeks, it is decided to institute a trial of subcutaneous hydration. This will be regularly reviewed according to its relative benefits and burdens, and according to Mary's overall condition.

Withdrawing and withholding treatment: cardiopulmonary resuscitation (CPR)

Cardiopulmonary resuscitation (CPR) can theoretically be attempted on every individual prior to death because failure of cardiac and respiratory function is part of dying. There is evidence to suggest that, for terminally ill patients, the harms of attempted CPR are likely by far to outweigh the benefits (George *et al*, 1989; Willard, 2000). The evidence indicates that, almost invariably, CPR either is unsuccessful or else re-establishes cardiopulmonary function for a very short time and a further cardiopulmonary arrest occurs during the same hospital admission.

The National Council for Hospice and Specialist Palliative Care Services (Joint working party between the National Council for Specialist Palliative Care Services and the Ethics Committee of the Association for Palliative Medicine of Great Britain and Ireland, 1997) has produced a document on CPR for people who are terminally ill. In summary, it states that there is no ethical obligation to carry out or discuss CPR with the majority of palliative care patients, for whom such treatment, following assessment, is judged to be futile. In the context of open discussion, raising such issues may be redundant and potentially distressing. It is important to recognise that this guidance does differ in some ways from that found in the joint statement published in the *Journal of Medical Ethics* (2001) by the BMA, the Resuscitation Council (UK) and the Royal College of Nursing (RCN) entitled, 'Decisions relating to cardiopulmonary resuscitation'.

If the likely outcome of a CPR intervention is uncertain, anticipatory decisions either to implement or withhold CPR should be sensitively explored with the patient. Both the likelihood of success and the resulting quality of life are appropriate issues for discussion. Decisions should be reviewed if the patient's clinical condition changes significantly. If a patient would likely benefit from CPR and also wishes for it, then it should be carried out in the event of cardiopulmonary arrest. Traditionally, hospices and social-care facilities have limited facilities for CPR. However, this need not stand as an obstacle to a patient's admission to such units, since a patient may accept admission on the understanding that initial resuscitative measures will be instituted, followed by transfer to a hospital equipped to undertake CPR.

Conclusion

Ethical decision-making at the end of life is often complex and challenging. Lack of previous experience, communication difficulties and varying levels of capacity all contribute to making such decision-making particularly difficult for the person with learning disability and for their carers. Professionals should have a good understanding of the medical, legal and ethical issues that might arise at this time so that they can provide support and guidance. They should also have mediation skills, and should be willing to hear and respect the opinions of family members and other carers. Above all, professionals should have the skills to enable the person with learning disability to play an active role in decision-making.

Dame Cicely Saunders made a promise to people facing death that is central to the philosophy of palliative care:

You matter because you are you. You matter to the last moment of your life, and we will do all we can, not only to help you die peacefully, but also to live until you die.

To achieve this goal for people with learning disabilities, it is our responsibility to participate in a compassionate and committed way when decisions are made on end-of-life issues. We should not be afraid of the complexity of these issues, but instead be willing to explore them and, if necessary, question our previous practice. Combining the expertise of both the palliative-care and learning-disability teams, and drawing on expert ethical guidance where available, is the best way to manage the end-of-life care of people with learning disabilities.

References

Airedale NHS Trust *vs* Bland [1993] 1 All ER 821

Aunos M, Feldman MA (2002) Attitudes towards sexuality, sterilization and parenting rights of persons with intellectual disabilities. *J Appl Res Intellect Disabil* **15**: 285–96

Beauchamp TL, Faden RR (1995) Informed consent: II. Meaning and elements of informed consent. In: Reich WT (ed) *Encyclopedia of Bioethics*. Rev edn. Vol 3. Simon & Schuster

Macmillan, New York

British Medical Association (1995) *Advance Statements*. BMJ Publishing Group, London

British Medical Association (2001) *Withholding and Withdrawing Life-prolonging Medical Treatment*. 2nd edn. BMJ Books, London

British Medical Association, Resuscitation Council (UK), Royal College of Nursing (2001) Decisions relating to cardiopulmonary resuscitation: a joint statement. *J Med Ethics* **27**: 310–6 (September 2001)

Brown H, Burns S, Flynn M (2002) *Supporting People through Terminal Illness and Death in Today and Tomorrow: the Report of the Growing Older with Learning Disabilities Programme*. The Foundation for People with Learning Disabilities, London

Canadian Healthcare Association, Canadian Medical Association, Canadian Nurses Association, Catholic Health Association of Canada (1999) *Joint Statement on Preventing and Resolving Ethical Conflicts Involving Health Care Providers and Persons Receiving Care*. CHA Press, Canada

Department for Constitutional Affairs (2004) *Mental Capacity Bill: Draft Code of Practice*. The Stationery Office, London

Department for Constitutional Affairs (2005) Mental Capacity Act. ISBN 0 10 540905 7. The Stationery Office, London

Doka K (2005) Ethics, end-of-life decisions and grief. *Mortality* **10**(1): 83–90

DPI (1982) *Proceedings of the First World Congress, Singapore: Disabled People's International*

Ellis PM, Tattershall MH (1999) How should doctors communicate the diagnosis of cancer to patients? *Ann Med* **31**(5): 336–41

General Medical Council (GMC) (2000) *Confidentiality: Protecting and Providing Information*. GMC, London

GMC (2002) *Withholding and Withdrawing Life-prolonging Treatments: Good Practice in Decision-making*. GMC, London

George AL, Folk BP, Crecelius PL (1989) Pre-arrest morbidity and other correlates of survival after in-hospital cardiopulmonary arrest. *Am J Med* **87**: 28–34

Gerle B, Lunden G, Sandblom P (1960) The patient with inoperable cancer from the psychiatric and social standpoints. *Cancer* **13**: 1206–17

Holloway D (2004) Ethical dilemmas in community learning disabilities nursing: what helps nurses resolve ethical dilemmas that result from choices made by people with learning disabilities? *J Learn Disabil* **8**(3): 283–98

Keywood K, Fovargue S, Flynn M (1999) *Best Practice? Healthcare Decision-making by, with and for Adults with Learning Disabilities*. NDT, Manchester

Law Commission of England and Wales (1995) Mental Incapacity (No. 231). Paragraph 3.3

Lord Chancellor's Department (2003a) *Making Decisions: Helping People who have Difficulty Deciding for Themselves. A Guide for People with Learning Difficulties*. The Stationery Office, London

Lord Chancellor's Department (2003b) *Making Decisions: Helping People who have Difficulty Deciding for Themselves. A Guide for Family and Friends*. The Stationery Office, London

Lord Chancellor's Department (2003c) *Making Decisions: Helping People who have Difficulty Deciding for Themselves. A Guide for Social Care Professionals*. The Stationery Office, London

Lord Chancellor's Department (2003d) *Making Decisions: Helping People who have Difficulty Deciding for Themselves. A Guide for Healthcare Professionals*. The Stationery Office, London

Lord Chancellor's Department (2003e) *Making Decisions: Helping People who have Difficulty Deciding for Themselves. A Guide for Legal Practitioners*. The Stationery Office, London

Lord Chancellor's Department (2004f) *Making Decisions: Helping People who have Difficulty Deciding for Themselves. Planning Ahead. A Guide for People who Wish to Plan for Possible Future Incapacity*. The Stationery Office, London

Lord Irvine of Lairg, The Lord Chancellor. *Who Decides? Making Decisions on Behalf of Mentally Incapacitated Adults. A Consultation Paper*. Issued by the Lord Chancellor's Department. Oral Statement to the House of Lords, Wednesday, 10 December, 1997

Lord Chancellor's Department (1997) *Who Decides? Making Decisions on Behalf of Mentally Incapacitated Adults* (Cm 3803). HMSO, London

McEnhill L (2004) Disability. In: Oliviere D, Monroe B (eds) *Death, Dying and Social Differences*. Oxford University Press, Oxford

National Council for Hospice and Specialist Palliative Care Services and Ethics Committee, Association for Palliative Medicine of Great Britain and Ireland Joint Working Party (1997) Ethical decision making in palliative care: artificial hydration for people who are terminally ill. *Eur J Palliat Care* **4**: 203–7

National Council for Hospice and Specialist Palliative Care Services and Ethics Committee, Association for Palliative Medicine of Great Britain and Ireland Joint Working Party (2002) *Ethical Decision Making in Palliative Care: Cardiopulmonary Resuscitation for People who are Terminally Ill*. National Council for Hospice and Specialist Palliative Care Services, London

NHS Cancer Screening Programme (2000) *Good Practice in Breast and Cervical Screening for Women with Learning Disabilities*. NHSCSP Publications, Sheffield

Northfield J, Turnbull J (2001) Experiences from cancer services. In: Hogg J *et al* (ed) *Cancer and People with Learning Disabilities: the Evidence from Published Studies and Experiences from Cancer Services*. BILD Publications, Kidderminster

Randall F, Downie RS (1999) *Palliative Care Ethics*. 2nd edn. Oxford University Press, Oxford

Tuffrey-Wijne I (1997) Palliative care and learning difficulties. *Nurs Times* **93**(31): 50–1

Tuffrey-Wijne I (2002) The palliative care needs of people with intellectual disabilities: a case study. *Int J Palliat Nurs* **8**(5): 222–32

Williams JR (2005) *World Medical Association Medical Ethics Manual*. The Medical Ethics Unit of the World Medical Association, Ferney-Voltaire Cedex

Willard C (2000) Cardiopulmonary resuscitation for palliative care patients: a discussion of ethical issues. *Palliat Med* **14**: 308–12

CHAPTER 7

Communication in the dying context

Sue Read

He dies and makes no sign.
   Shakespeare, *Henry VI*, 3.3.29

Communication involves the sharing of meaningful interactions with other people. Communication theory explores the processes that are inherent in communication, namely 'the selection of a means of conveying a message (language, gesture, writing), the decoding of the message by the recipient (hearing, seeing, reading), and making a response on the basis of the interpretation (reply)' (Randall and Parker, 2000: 69). Effective communication skills are often seen as the core skills of helping relationships (Parkes, Relf and Couldrick, 1996), particularly in palliative and terminal care contexts. Many people with learning disabilities have difficulties in communication, which may affect how they express their needs and wants to others, and indeed how others respond to such needs and wants in a variety of care contexts. This chapter aims to identify the issues involved in communicating with people with learning disabilities who are dying. Once identified, such challenges will be explored and strategies offered to promote the sharing of meaningful interactions, thereby improving clinical effectiveness within this sensitive area.

Vulnerable people

The Department of Health (DoH) describe people with learning disabilities as having a reduced ability to understand new or complex information, or to learn new skills (impaired intelligence) with a reduced ability to cope independently (impaired social functioning), which started before adulthood and with a lasting effect on development (DoH, 2001). This functional definition promotes people first and foremost as individuals and emphasises their strengths and abilities rather than their limitations. The DoH (2001: 14) goes on to say that, 'People with learning disability are amongst the most socially excluded and vulnerable groups in Britain today'. People with learning disabilities who are dying may be described as particularly vulnerable, as a direct result of their intellectual disability and their palliative illness. They are perceived as experiencing 'double jeopardy when it comes to having their needs met and their rights and entitlement to proper treatment and palliative health care honoured' (Read and Elliot, 2003).

About twenty people per thousand have learning disabilities in the UK; of these, three to four per thousand will have severe or profound learning disabilities (O'Hara and Sperlinger, 1997). The DoH (2001) suggests that the number of people with learning disabilities may increase by around 1% per annum over the next fifteen years. This is a result of an increased life expectancy (particularly among people with Down syndrome); a growing number of children and young people with complex and multiple disabilities who are now surviving into adulthood; a sharp rise in the number of school-age children with autistic spectrum disorders (some of whom will have a learning disability); and a greater prevalence among some minority ethnic populations of South Asian origin (DoH, 2001). Consequently, for those people who present with a variety of learning disabilities, now physically integrated into mainstream society, a range of services (both voluntary and statutory) needs to be developed in response to the specialist needs and requirements of this growing population. Such services include palliative care.

With rapid advances in health care, people with learning disabilities are living longer, and will inevitably experience the deaths of members of their family and friends. Yet, as Oswin (2000: 31) writes: 'despite all the advances made in changing attitudes towards people with learning difficulties, it appears that in the area of loss and bereavement they are still not receiving enough consideration, nor the appropriate support they require'. People with learning disabilities are a minority, disadvantaged and devalued group; they are often perceived as child-like in terms of their cognition, abilities and physical support needs; and they are frequently treated paternalistically — over-protected and shielded from painful experiences such as death, dying and bereavement.

'People with developmental disabilities function on a developmental level that is inconsistent with their chronological age' (Lavin, 2002: 314). If death comprehension is to be more associated with cognition rather than chronological age in people with learning disabilities, and life experiences important in enhancing understanding of death and bereavement, then it is crucial that people with learning disabilities can actively participate in death, dying and bereavement in order to learn how to cope with such events. Consequently, people with learning disabilities need to be exposed to the pain of death and bereavement in a sensitive, constructive and supportive way. However, this may not always be the case. People with learning disabilities, for a variety of reasons, continue to be excluded from death, dying and bereavement. Communication remains a key element within theses issues.

Disenfranchised grief

Generally, bereaved people have a perceived sense of disempowerment after bereavement. For people with a learning disability, this sense of disempowerment is often total, as both personal and professional carers try to protect them from the full impact of the loss (Elliot, 1995) and learning-disabled people are actively discouraged from being involved in the process of death, dying and its aftermath (ie. bereavement). Carers may often be uncertain about how to handle grief because of the potential for varied reactions (Thurm, 1989) and sometimes may not feel skilled enough to offer adequate support.

Many people with learning disabilities are still being denied the opportunity to participate in bereavement rituals, despite the identified increased risk of psychiatric problems when they are excluded from doing so (Oswin, 1985, 1991). Raji and Hollins (2003) conducted a multicultural study in an inner-London borough to examine local religious and cultural practices following the bereavement of people with learning disabilities. Semi-structured interviews were done with six funeral directors and representatives from three religious groups to establish local practices, resources and knowledge. They found that people with learning disabilities are still socially excluded from bereavement and funeral rituals, although some funeral directors had adapted their premises to accommodate the physical needs of these people.

According to Oswin (1991), bereaved people with learning disabilities may often be denied the time or privacy required to deal with their grief, and changes in behaviour or mood may go unnoticed by carers. Ray (1978) found that the true intensity of grief was unexpected by parents of people with learning disabilities and Strachen (1981) described the difficulties that nurses had in knowing if the people in their care understood the finality of loss. Because clients are not able to make their needs known, and are not actively involved in bereavement, this may result in grief responses often being delayed (Kitching, 1987). She also asserted that cognition and emotional expression were not linked. However, the ability of some people with learning disabilities to express their grief in a socially acceptable manner may prove difficult.

Rothenberg (1994) described the impact of bereavement on emotional health because of the developmental disability itself and the lack of appropriate psychological preparation for death. Carers may not know how to address the issues of bereaved people with multiple, complex needs, and may be fearful of a difficult response from those people with a history of challenging behaviours. Such thinking provides erroneous excuses to protect carers from having to address difficult issues (such as death and dying), either personally or professionally.

Read and Elliot (2003) argued that if you have a learning disability, you are likely to be involved in death and dying less than other non-disabled people; if you have a learning disability and additional associated sensory or physical disabilities, you are even less likely to be actively involved; and if you have challenging behaviours, you stand even less chance of being involved. Such additional disabilities serve to increase dependency on others and reduce active engagement in difficult situations such as death, dying and bereavement. Clearly, people with learning disabilities are extremely vulnerable, reliant on so many people for so much help.

Active exclusion from the process of death has been powerfully and articulately described by Doka (1989) as disenfranchised grief, and the author views this work as being pivotal to an understanding of the lack of active involvement in the grief process (Read, 1999). Doka described disenfranchised grief as 'the grief that persons experience when they incur a loss that cannot be openly acknowledged, publicly mourned, or socially supported' (1989: 4). Initially, he identified three reasons for this disenfranchisement:

1. The relationship to the deceased is not recognised (where the relationship between the bereaved and the deceased is not based on recognisable kin ties).
2. The loss is not recognised (where the loss itself is not socially defined as significant).
3. Finally, the griever is not recognised (where the person is not socially defined as capable of grief).

More recently, Doka (2002) has added two further factors: the circumstances surrounding the death (such as suicide) and the ways that individuals grieve (eg. styles of grieving and cultural factors). These factors often result in a lack of inclusion in any associated ritual, for example, attending the funeral, which, as Doka reminds us, is often perceived as a service of the living and which is only acknowledged for those who are thought of as being 'legitimate' mourners, or grief sanctioned by society. Marginalised groups, such as people with learning disability, frequently do not have their grief legitimised by society, and attendance at funerals, for example, continues to be difficult for this population (Raji and Hollins, 2003).

Doka (1989) argued that the very nature of disenfranchised grief created extra problems for grievers. Whilst removing or minimising sources of support, he suggested that for many disenfranchised grievers, such as children and people with learning disabilities, there were no coherent, well-organised or readily available support systems to help them. Doka further asserted that responses to grief can therefore be complicated for the disenfranchised griever.

Disenfranchised death

Whilst Doka's (1989, 2003) concept of disenfranchised grief is important in relation to those survivors of death who may be socially excluded from the rituals associated with the dead, people with learning disabilities may also experience disenfranchised death, when confronted by their own impending death, for a number of reasons. When a death can be anticipated (for example, where there has been a palliative illness), this is usually experienced as a sudden death by the person with learning disability, since he or she is rarely told in advance of the event (O'Nians, 1993; see *Case Study 7.1: Jane and David*).

Such paternalistic attitudes and over-protectiveness exclude the individual with a learning disability from being actively involved with their dying relatives and from saying their 'goodbyes' in a meaningful way. Sudden death is regarded as being one of life's most difficult deaths to accommodate because of its complexity and nature (Wright, 1991). Yet, well-meaning carers often burden people with sudden death because of the difficulties involved in preparing them (or anticipating) the death when possible. Such unhelpful responses are still common.

Disenfranchised death can be described as death that is not openly acknowledged with the dying person, where the dying person is socially excluded from the process of dying and deliberately excluded from the decision-making processes surrounding the terminal illness. Disenfranchised death involves several features (*Panel 7.1*).

Case Study 7.1: Jane and David

Jane and David had been married for eleven years when David was eventually diagnosed with inoperable lung cancer. They both had a learning disability, worked in sheltered employment (part-time) and lived together in a flat.

As David's condition deteriorated, he was finally admitted to a local nursing home. When explaining about the seriousness of his illness, nurses talked to David's wife about him 'not getting better'. This is significantly different than saying that he was going to die of his illness, and was very confusing to Jane.

Similarly, the nursing staff were reluctant to tell David himself that he was going to die because they felt uncertain as to how he would cope with the news.

> ## Panel 7.1: Features of disenfranchised death
>
> - The autonomy of the dying person is not recognised (where the person is not socially defined as capable of comprehending their own mortality).
> - The pending death is not recognised or legitimised with the person dying (the person is not told or prepared for his or her own death).
> - The person's 'rights to know' are overlooked (as carers struggle with the ability to communicate in a meaningful way).
> - The circumstances surrounding the death (i.e. the nature and context of pending death); communication challenges; and the ability of the terminally ill person to comprehend the concept of death (cognition) may contribute cumulatively to the disenfranchised features illustrated.

Whilst these factors may protect the carers from the challenges of confronting the dying person with difficult issues, questions, options and choices, they also ensure that the person with learning disability has no control whatsoever over what is happening to him or her in the latter stages of life. Disenfranchised death, like disenfranchised grief, may be experienced by a range of marginalised groups including children; the elderly; people with mental health problems; and people with learning disabilities. Many of the disenfranchising effects are related to the attitudes, beliefs and values towards 'different-ness' in society generally, and carers specifically. However, the challenges of effective communication are important factors.

Addressing communication challenges

Since more than half of people with learning disabilities may present with some form of communication impairment (Kerr *et al*, 1996), then communicating in a meaningful way may be challenging to many carers, and never more so than in the palliative care context. Sensory impairments are often associated with learning disability (Hodges, 2003), and people who have profound and complex needs may be unable to use language in any form (eg. speech, signing or symbols). They are likely to be communicating at a very basic level (Ware, 1997, cited in Porter et al, 2001), involving signals such as reflex responses, actions, sounds and facial expression. Working with people with such complex needs requires the carers to acquire a variety and flexible range of communication skills, which can involve touch, music and singing (Hodges, 2003). From a palliative care perspective, communication will be particularly important in areas such as: recognising ill-health; talking about illness and death; breaking bad news; and talking with others about difficult topics (Read, 1998a).

Recognising ill-health

The DoH (1995) advocates that 'people with learning disabilities should have access to all general health services, including health promotion and health education, and primary and secondary

---

Panel 7.2: Difficulties in recognising ill-health in people with learning disabilities (after Read, 2003)

- The symptoms may not be easily identified, recognised or acknowledged.
- Diagnostic overshadowing, where symptoms are perceived as being part of the learning disability (Brown et al, 2003).
- The seriousness of the illness may be trivialised or ignored.
- Lack of attendance at health-screening and health-promotion clinics.
- Families and carers may not have the necessary skills or knowledge to support the individual with a learning disability in obtaining appropriate treatment or in the maintenance of health-related behaviour (Howells, 1997).
- Individuals may have difficulties communicating their discomfort or experiences of severe pain (Keenan and McIntosh, 2000).
- Individuals may be treated by some health and social care professionals as passive recipients (Keenan and McIntosh, 2000).
- Poor communication channels may exist between individuals, organisations and professional disciplines.

---

health care with appropriate additional support to meet these needs'. Unfortunately, many people with learning disabilities have healthcare needs that may go unnoticed, and consequently untreated, until well-advanced; hence, it may be too late for the individual to respond to curative treatment (Tuffrey-Wijne, 1997). Carers may have difficulties in recognising ill-health amongst people with learning disabilities (*Panel 7.2*).

Pain assessment and recognition may be generally difficult because of the complexities of its biological and psychological components (Jones, 2003). Self-reporting of pain remains an important feature of pain-management (Jones, 2003) and some individuals with learning disabilities may have great difficulties in both recognising their own pain and making their distress known in a socially acceptable and meaningful way.

Carers have a pivotal role in identifying distress in clients who are limited in their ability to communicate in any conventional manner, since any behavioural change — new behaviours; absence of usual behaviours; increased frequency or intensity of existing behaviours — may be an indicator of innate distress. The pain and symptom management of this client population may incorporate a host of challenges, many of which are addressed in *Chapter 4*.

Within palliative care generally, studies have suggested a correlation between good communication and psychological well-being (Bishara *et al*, 1997; May, 1993), but nurse-patient communication skills still prove problematic. Challenges to effective communication may include the professionals' perceived lack of skills; professional fears (of upsetting the patient; of unleashing strong emotions); and patients' fears, attitudes and beliefs (Heaven and Maguire, 2003). From a learning-disability perspective, problems in communication may arise from the learning disability itself (and any associated sensory impairments); environmental or organisational factors; and the prevailing negative attitudes associated with the disability (Ingram, 1991). The learning disability itself may constitute a whole range of thinking and reasoning difficulties (Conboy-Hill, 1991) that affect the person's ability to articulate in a clear, meaningful fashion. Effective communication is vital in identifying and responding appropriately to ill-health in people with learning disabilities.

Time is an important consideration for good communication, as some people with learning disabilities may have limited attention span, limited abstract abilities (Conboy-Hill, 1991) and may need information to be repeated frequently and in different forms (perhaps using books or photographs). Such approaches are often both labour- and time-intensive.

Health promotion involves helping the individual to become more aware of their own bodies and of the importance of recognising and talking about any changes, since this can help any illness be diagnosed more readily. For example, women with learning disabilities may have 'fragmented access' to breast-screening services (Symonds and Howsam, 2004), but books such as *Looking After My Breasts* (Hollins and Perez, 2000) and *Keeping Healthy Down Below* (Hollins and Downer, 2000) may be useful in translating important issues into easier, accessible formats. Additionally, the DoH (2000) guidelines, *Good Practice in Breast and Cervical Screening for Women with Learning Disabilities*, support professional carers to help women access regular and appropriate screening.

Group work has been identified as a useful vehicle from which to explore sensitive topics with adults with learning disabilities (Read *et al*, 2000). Proactive educational groups would encourage people to talk openly about issues related to self-image, body image, illness, loss and changes in the body. They would also make people feel more comfortable when talking about potentially embarrassing issues, including those surrounding ill-health.

Talking about ill-health

A key issue in palliative care is that of breaking bad news. Buckman (1984) describes bad news as any news that drastically and negatively alters the patient's perception of his or her future. Although diagnosis, prognosis and treatment options all carry the potential to involve bad news to differing degrees, death is often perceived as the ultimate bad news, perhaps because of its negative impact, permanence and irreversibility (Read and Jervis, 2003). Kaye (1995) argues that bad news needs to be broken effectively in order to:

- Maintain trust between patients and professionals.
- Reduce uncertainty.
- Allow appropriate adjustment so that the patient can make informed judgement.
- Prevent a conspiracy of silence, which may destroy family communication and prevent mutual support (Kaye, 1995).

Breaking bad news may carry a range of personal, professional and social challenges (Buckman, 1991). When it involves people with learning disabilities, it is often accompanied by additional considerations, as professional carers endeavour to overcome a host of attitudinal, cognitive and complex communication challenges associated with the learning disability itself (Read, 1998b). Buckman's six-step protocol (1991) is a useful framework for supporting those involved in breaking bad news generally, and particularly when it involves people with learning disability (Read, 1998b). Although 'there may be no right words for breaking bad news' (Faulkner, 1998: 13), there can be a set of principles or guidelines in the form of a protocol that can help the professional deliver the news in a sensitive and meaningful way (Maguire *et al*, 1995). *Figure*

Figure 7.1: A model to promote communication when breaking difficult news.

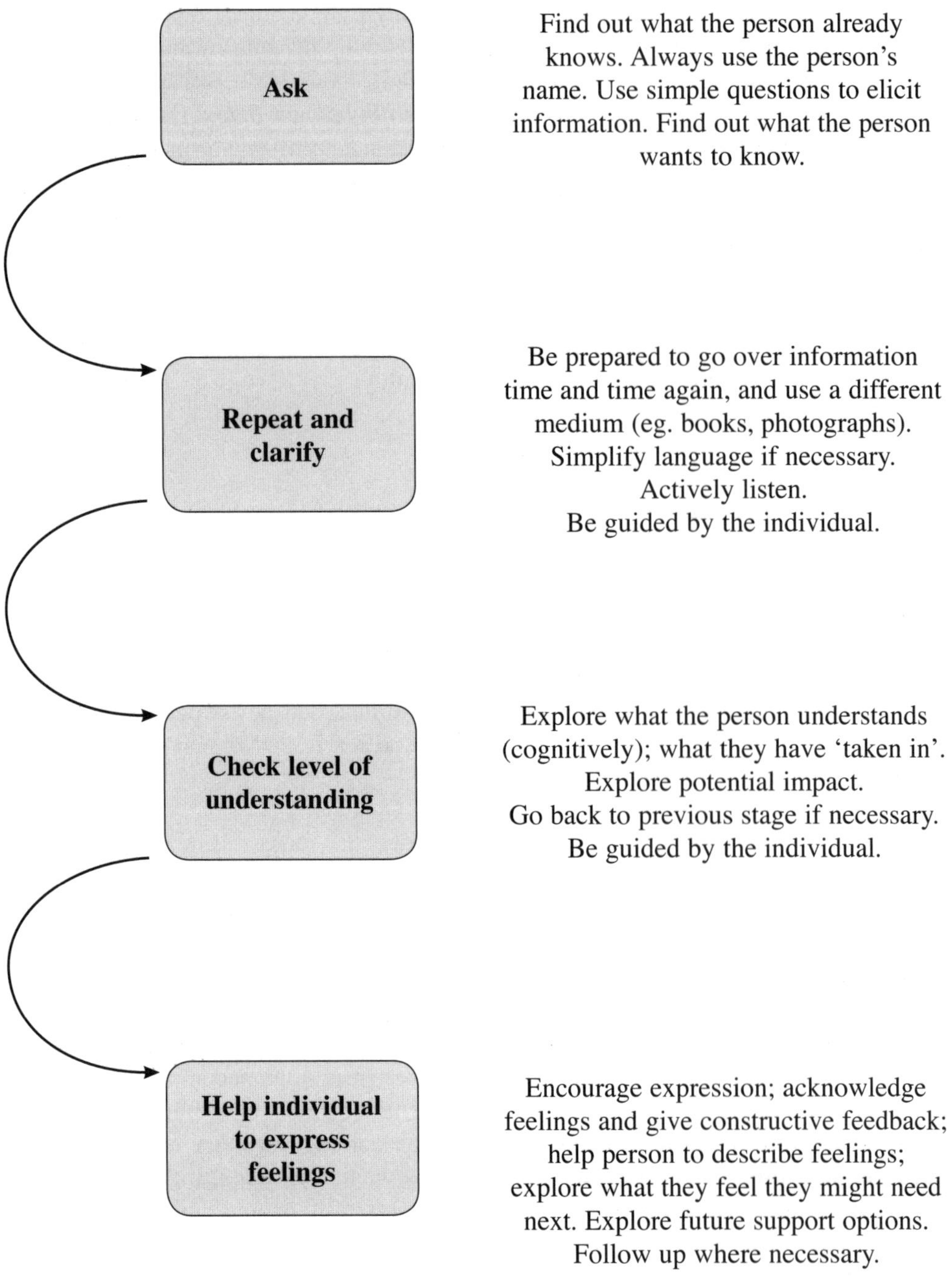

Ask

Find out what the person already knows. Always use the person's name. Use simple questions to elicit information. Find out what the person wants to know.

Repeat and clarify

Be prepared to go over information time and time again, and use a different medium (eg. books, photographs). Simplify language if necessary. Actively listen. Be guided by the individual.

Check level of understanding

Explore what the person understands (cognitively); what they have 'taken in'. Explore potential impact. Go back to previous stage if necessary. Be guided by the individual.

Help individual to express feelings

Encourage expression; acknowledge feelings and give constructive feedback; help person to describe feelings; explore what they feel they might need next. Explore future support options. Follow up where necessary.

7.1 presents a similar framework for communicating bad news to people with learning disabilities specifically. The ARCH — Ask, Repeat, Check, Help — model offers a simple framework from which to develop a therapeutic dialogue in relation to bad news.

Both verbal and non-verbal communication are important components in communication theory (Randall and Parker, 2000). Touch and physical contact have been described as 'a language of relationships: a language allowing the carer to communicate a healing message to those who may be struggling in doubt, loneliness and fear' (Autton, 1996: 123). Language can be accompanied by touch, and for some people who have multiple and complex needs, touch may be the only form of communication with the outside world. The ability to communicate effectively may deteriorate as the palliative illness progresses, and holding the hand of a dying patient or placing a comforting arm around a person's shoulder lets them know that you are there, and conveys a positive message that you are trying to communicate with them on a human level.

However, the carer has to feel comfortable when using touch with a dying person, in order for it to be effective (Autton, 1996).

Explaining treatments may be difficult and books such as *Getting on with Cancer* (Donaghey *et al*, 2002), which make good use of simple pictures to explain complex procedures (eg. radiotherapy, chemotherapy, X-rays) in simple ways, can enhance communication. For some patients, perhaps a visit to the clinic to view the equipment (perhaps take photographs if appropriate) and rehearse the procedure may be a viable option worth exploring.

Communication is a complex issue; *Panel 7.3* offers a range of suggestions that serve to improve communication and minimise the barriers to reciprocal and meaningful support, particularly in the palliative care context.

Some people with a learning disability may need an open invitation (or even permission) to talk about difficult topics, such as death and dying. Similarly, familiar carers need to feel comfortable talking about, and exploring feelings associated with, death and dying, and education will be important in preparing carers to handle difficult topics and discussions. Multidisciplinary training or education (around such topics as coping with loss and grief, how to offer an invitation to talk and dealing with sensitive issues) can offer valuable preparation.

Panel 7.3: Addressing communication challenges

- A familiar person should be actively involved whenever possible.
- Allow time for the person to inspect and digest new information, either verbally or visually.
- Use visual stimuli such as pictures, books, photographs and cue cards, together with short and simple sentences, to help improve understanding and recall.
- Break tasks down into smaller, more easily understandable tasks (Ambula, 1977).
- Use creative media such as drawing, painting, modelling, music, drama and poetry to elicit feelings and emotions (Read, 1999).
- Use language that is simple and concrete.
- Vary the ways in which information is given (eg. verbally and/or visually).
- Record information on audiotape so that individuals can take it with them.
- Involve the individual as much as possible in his or her illness, subsequent treatment options (or not), and eventual death.

Talking with others about difficult topics

Death never occurs in a 'vacuum', but within a unique, social context. When a person with a learning disability dies, friends, family and carers may grieve for the person who has died, and miss them in their own particular fashion. When the friends of the deceased also have learning disability, there is a tendency to shield them from the anticipated death and protect them from the reality, sadness and impact of death when it eventually occurs.

When a person is dying, it may be helpful to include friends who live with them in the natural, dying process. Isolating the dying person perpetuates the pervading mystery and secrecy around death and dying. Carers should try actively to involve any friends who live in the home within the dying process, should the friends want this. This might involve simply encouraging friends to sit with the terminally ill person, perhaps to listen to music together; to collect a cup from the bedroom; to take fresh linen; or to take some flowers. Encourage friends to see the person who is ill, so that they can appreciate how ill the person really is. This confrontation with 'concrete' reality may encourage the friends to talk about the illness and ask difficult, but necessary, questions, such as, 'Is he going to die?'). Such sensitive exposure will also prepare them for the inevitable death, when it occurs.

Carers also need to anticipate difficult decisions in preparation for the death, which could helpfully be discussed as part of the care team. Such issues might involve questions such as:

- how might we break the news of the death?
- who might be the most appropriate person to break the news?
- what sort of language might be needed?
- will friends want to see the person after death?
- will friends want to visit the Chapel of Rest?
- which friends would want to go to the funeral?

Seeing a person who has died in his or her own bed may be less traumatic than seeing someone in a coffin at the Chapel of Rest. However, some people may misinterpret the bed and associate it with the person simply 'being asleep' rather than dead, and may need to see him or her in both contexts. Using simple, concrete and consistent language remains important throughout, and all carers should use the same words (eg. 'dead') to promote understanding and reinforce the finality and irreversibility of death. When preparing people to view a dead body, carers should try to explain exactly what they might see, smell, feel and hear. For example, carers should explain that:

- the body will be lying flat (in a bed or a wooden box called a 'coffin')
- the person cannot move, hear, see, breathe, eat or speak
- the body will be cold to the touch
- the body will look a different colour
- there may be music playing in the background
- there may be a musty smell of incense burning.

Dealing with death and dying may affect professional carers in various ways, as Worden (1991: 133–4) points out:

1. It makes us aware of our own losses.
2. It makes us aware of our potential losses.
3. It makes us aware of our own mortality.

Although prepared for the death, carers may find this time very traumatic and need to be able to access extra support and advice from specialists in this field (such as a bereavement organisation, hospices and the clergy) for practical help and advice, and supervision for personal support. Communicating these needs are also important.

Conclusion

It appears that, as with non-disabled individuals, responses to death and grief are numerous and varied among people with learning disabilities. Associated carers need to have a repertoire of skills and approaches to deal with such responses in a way that is meaningful to, and appropriate for, the individual. For some individuals, the need for a more specialist intervention (ie. a bereavement counsellor) may be required (Elliot, 1995; Read *et al*, 1999; Read, 2001).

People with learning disabilities, for a variety of both obvious and erroneous reasons, continue to be excluded from death, dying and bereavement. They are also described as having an external locus of control, dependent on others for (for example) care needs and decisions about care options, particularly involving death and bereavement. Arthur (2003) acknowledged that, despite the considerable attention paid to describing and addressing cognitive functioning, service planning and evaluation, the emotional needs of people with learning disabilities have remained largely neglected. He suggested that 'the challenge throws up our own disability when confronted with complex behaviour that cannot be easily understood, communicated or treated in conventional ways' (2003: 28). Such challenges have influenced how, and indeed if, people with learning disabilities have had their losses acknowledged and have subsequently been involved in death, dying and bereavement. The concept of disenfranchised grief (Doka, 1989, 2003) has been explicitly linked to disenfranchised death to reflect the inherent difficulties that are often present when people with learning disabilities are faced with their own pending mortality. Communication remains a central feature to providing appropriate holistic care and support in the palliative context.

Whilst people with learning disabilities have more similarities to, rather than differences from, people who have a palliative illness generally, they may have additional issues (largely related to their disability directly, and other associated impairments) that affect: how and when an individual's illness is diagnosed; what treatment options are available and accessible; and the individual's autonomy and empowerment within the palliative care journey. The attitudes of carers remain influential, and communication within this process will remain important if individuals with a learning disability are to be actively involved in death, dying and bereavement. More research is required by the clinicians involved to clarify the issues and explore effective communication with this population in this complex sphere of care.

Sue Read

References

Ambula S (1997) Communication. In: O'Hara J, Sperlinger A (eds) (1997) *Adults with Learning Disabilities: a Practical Approach for Healthcare Professionals*. Wiley & Sons, Chichester

Arthur AR (2003) The emotional lives of people with learning disability. *Br J Learn Disabil* **31**: 25–30

Autton N (1996) The use of touch in palliative care. *Eur J Palliat Care* **3**(3): 121–4

Bishara E, Loew F, Forest MI, Fabre J, Baro V (1997) Is there a relationship between psychological well-being and patient-carer consensus? A clinical pilot study. *J Palliat Care* **13**: 14–22

Brown H, Burns S, Flynn M (2003) 'Please don't let it happen on my shift!': supporting staff who are caring for people with learning disabilities who are dying. *Tizard Learn Disabil Rev* **8**(2): 32–41

Buckman R (1984) Why breaking bad news is difficult. In: R Buckman (ed) (1991). *How to Break Bad News: a Guide for Healthcare Professionals*. Papermac, London

Buckman R (1991) *How to Break Bad News: a Guide for Healthcare Professionals*. Papermac, London

Conboy-Hill S (1992) Grief, loss and people with learning disabilities. In: Waitman A, Conboy-Hill S (eds) *Psychotherapy and Mental Handicap*. Sage, London

DoH (1995) *The Health of the Nation: Strategy for People with Learning Disabilities*. DoH, London

DoH (2000) *Good Practice in Breast and Cervical Screening for Women with Learning Disabilities*. NHS Cancer Screening Programme, Sheffield

DoH (2001a) *Valuing People: a New Strategy for Learning Disability for the 21ˢᵗ Century*. DoH, London

Doka KJ (ed) (1989) *Disenfranchised Grief: Recognising Hidden Sorrow*. Lexington, Lexington (MA)

Doka KJ (ed) (2002) *Disenfranchised Grief: New Directions, Challenges and Strategies for Practice*. Research Press, Illinois

Donaghey V, Bernat J, Tuffrey-Wijne I, Hollins S (2002) *Getting on with Cancer*. Gaskell/St George's Hospital Medical School, London

Elliot D (1995) Helping people with learning disabilities to handle grief. *Nurs Times* **91**(43): 27–9

Faulkner A (1998) *When the News is Bad: a Guide for Health Professionals*. Stanley Thornes, Cheltenham

Heaven C, Maguire P (2003) Communication issues. In: Lloyd-Williams M (ed) (2003) *Psychosocial Issues in Palliative Care*. OUP, Oxford

Hodges S (2003) *Counselling Adults with Learning Disabilities*. Palgrave Macmillan, Basingstoke

Hollins S, Perez W (2000) *Looking After My Breasts*. Gaskell & St George's Hospital Medical

104

School, London

Hollins S, Downer J (2000) *Keeping Healthy 'Down Below'*. Gaskell & St George's Hospital Medical School, London

Howells G (1997) A general practitioner perspective. In: O'Hara J, Sperlinger A (eds) (1997) *Adults with Learning Disabilities: a Practical Approach for Healthcare Professionals*. Wiley & Sons, Chichester

Hussain F, Raczeka R (1997) Life story work for people with learning disabilities. *Br J Learn Disabil* **25**(2): 73–6

Ingram R (1991) Learning difficulties and communication. *Nurs Stand* **5**(31): 36–9

Jones D (2003) Pain management and people with learning disabilities. *J Learn Disabil* **7**(4): 291–5

Kaye P (1995) *Breaking Bad News: a Ten-Step Approach*. EPL, Northampton

Keenan P, Macintosh P (2000) Learning disabilities and palliative care. *Palliat Care Today* **9**(1): 11–13

Kerr M, Fraser W, Felce D (1996) Primary healthcare for people with a learning disability. *Br J Learn Disabil* **24**(1): 2–8

Kitching N (1987) Helping people with mental handicaps cope with bereavement: a case study with discussion. *Ment Handicap* **15**: 60–3

Maguire P, Faulkner A, Regnard C (1995) Breaking bad news: a flow diagram. In: Regnard C, Hockley J (eds) *Flow Diagram in Advanced Cancer and Other Diseases*. Edward Arnold, London. Cited in: Faulkner A (1998) *When the News is Bad: a Guide for Health Professionals*. Stanley Thornes, Cheltenham

May C (1993) Subjectivity and culpability in the constitution of nurse-patient relationships. *Int J Nurs Stud* **39**(2): 181–92

O'Hara J, Sperlinger A (eds) (1997) *Adults with Learning Disabilities: a Practical Approach for Healthcare Professionals*. Wiley & Sons, Chichester

O'Nians R (1993) Support in grief. *Nurs Times* **89**(50): 624–5

Oswin M (1991) *Am I Allowed to Cry?* Souvenir Press, London

Oswin M (1991) *Am I Allowed to Cry?* 2nd edn. Souvenir Press, London

Parkes CM, Relf M, Couldrick A (1996) *Counselling in Terminal Care and Bereavement*. British Psychological Society, Leicester

Porter J, Ouvrey C, Morgan M, Downs C (2001) Interpreting the communication of people with profound and multiple learning difficulties. *Br J Learn Disabil* **29**: 12–16

Raji O, Hollins S (2003) How far are people with learning disabilities involved in funeral rites? *Br J Learn Disabil* **31**: 42–5

Randall P, Parker J (2000) Communication theory. In: Davies M (ed) (2000) *The Blackwell Encyclopaedia of Social Work*. Blackwell, Oxford

Read S (1998a) The palliative care needs of people with learning disabilities. *Int J Palliat Nurs* **4**(5): 246–51

Read S (1998b) Breaking bad news to people with a learning disability. *Br J Nurs* **7**(2): 86–91

Read S (1999) Creative ways of working when exploring the bereavement counselling process. In: Blackman N (ed) (1999) *Living with Loss: Helping People with Learning Disabilities Cope with Bereavement and Loss.* Pavilion Publishing, Brighton

Read S, Frost I, Messenger N, Oates S (1999) Bereavement counselling and support for people with a learning disability: identifying issues and exploring possibilities. *Br J Learn Disabil* **27**(3): 99–104

Read S, Papakosta-Harvey V, Bower S (2001) Using workshops on loss for adults with learning disabilities. *Groupwork* **12**(2): 6–26

Read S (2001) A year in the life of a bereavement counselling and support service for people with learning disabilities. *J Learn Disabil* **5**(1): 19–33

Read S (2003) Bereavement and loss. In: Markwick A, Parrish A (eds) (2003) *Learning Disabilities: Themes and Perspectives.* Butterworth Heinemann, Oxford

Read S, Elliot D (2003) Death and learning disability: a vulnerability perspective. *J Adult Protect* **5**(1): 5–13

Read S, Jervis J (2003) Sudden death. In: Wood I, Rhodes M (eds) (2003) *Medical Assessment Units: the Initial Management of Acute Medical Patients.* Whurr, London

Strachen JG (1981) Reactions to bereavement: a study of a group of adult mentally handicapped hospitalised residents. APEX. *J Br Instit Ment Handicap* **9**(1): 221

Sumonds D, Howsam K (2004) Breast awareness in learning disabilities. *Cancer Nurs Pract* **3**(1): 8–10

Thurm A (1989) I've lost a good friend. *Nurs Times* **85**(32): 66–8

Tuffrey-Wijne I (1997) Palliative care and people with learning disabilities. *Nurs Times* **93**(31): 50–1

Ware J (2001) Creating a responsive environment for people with profound and multiple leaning difficulties. In: Porter J, Ouvrey C, Morgan M, Downs C (2001) Interpreting the communication of people with profound and multiple learning difficulties. *Br J Learn Disabil* **2**: 12–16

Worden WJ (1991) *Grief Counselling and Grief Therapy: a Handbook for the Mental Health Practitioner.* 2nd edn. Routledge, London

Wright B (1991) *Sudden Death: Intervention Skills for the Caring Professions.* Churchill Livingstone, London

CHAPTER 8

Counselling and support

Sue Read

Arthur (2003) recognised that, despite considerable attention being paid to describing and addressing needs associated with cognitive functioning, service planning and evaluation, the emotional needs of people with learning disabilities remain largely neglected. There has been relatively little research published around counselling, psychotherapy and people with learning disabilities, which specifically focuses on the impact or outcomes of such approaches or that particularly relates to experiences involving bereavement or those faced with a life-limiting illness. There are also proportionately fewer empirical studies of counselling and psychotherapy involving people with learning disabilities compared with the wealth of literature around the topic areas generally. According to Hodges (2003), this may be due to: a general lack of knowledge about the emotional world of this client population; a pervasive belief that feelings are not relevant in understanding people with learning disabilities; the historical features of 'invisibility' and segregation of people with learning disabilities; negative stereotypes; the lack of prestige in working with learning disability; the difficulties in using standardised surveys and interviews; the challenges of gaining informed consent; and the difficulties of finding and using control groups for research purposes. Additionally, most outcome measures used in psychotherapy are in self-reporting formats, requiring average reading ability (Beail, 1995), which require creative redrafting to be appropriate for people with limited cognition and functional capacities. However, counselling as a means of support has been used with people with learning disabilities in a variety of differing contexts (Badelt, 1990; Portner, 1990; Strohmer and Prout, 1994; Read *et al*, 1999; Read, 2001; Hawkins, 2002; Hodges, 2003).

From a bereavement perspective, the need for grief-processing interventions, together with the need for factual information, meaningful ritual involvement and opportunities for talking and sharing, have been identified by both Kauffman (1994) and James (1995). Both researchers encouraged individuals to talk about the death, discuss the associated details and encouraged them to participate in the rituals surrounding the death. They also explored practical issues (eg. wheelchair access to churches) and the importance of keeping personal mementoes of the deceased. People with learning disabilities are described as wanting to share their emotions openly and directly, together with experiences of loss, death and dying (French and Kuczaj, 1992; McDaniel, 1989; Read and Papakosta-Harvey, 2004; Bower, 2001) and professional carers need to explore more constructive ways of helping them do this.

This chapter initially aims to introduce the concept of psychosocial support in palliative care, and to explore this concept, particularly in relation to the emotional needs of people with a learning disability. It will explore counselling as support and identify the need for flexible approaches when working in a person-centred way with this particular population.

Psychosocial support in palliative care

Supportive care is described by Jeffrey (2003) as care designed to support the patient and family in coping with the treatments involved in the palliative care journey. Jeffrey (2003) affirmed the key principles underpinning good supportive care as involving:

- a focus on quality of life
- a holistic approach
- care to include the patient and those who matter to the patient
- respect for autonomy and choice
- an emphasis on open and sensitive communication.

(Jeffrey, 2003: 4)

Within this, psychosocial support is a key element. The National Council for Hospice and Specialist Palliative Care Services (NCHSPCS, 1997; cited in Jeffrey, 2003: 3) defines psychosocial care as being:

> *… concerned with the psychological and emotional well-being of the patient and their family/carers, including issues of self-esteem, insight into adaptation of the illness and its consequences, communication, social functioning and relationships.*

The importance of psychological distress within palliative care is well-recognised (eg. Derogates *et al*, 1983; Maguire *et al*, 1978; Maguire *et al*, 1980; Walker *et al*, 2003), but not particularly from a learning-disability perspective. Therefore, there remains much to explore about the psychological support needs of people with a learning disability and their families, and how such needs can be best met, in the palliative care context.

According to Jeffrey (2003), good psychosocial care involves a holistic assessment of the patient, family and carer's needs, and this will involve assessing:

- the impact of the illness (on relationships and self-image)
- familiar coping strategies
- sources of support
- hopes and expectations
- perceived losses (previous, current and future)
- the meaning of the illness (to the patient and family)
- the patient's hopes and fears for the future.

(Jeffrey, 2003: 7)

Such an assessment would indicate the need for practical, emotional, psychological, social and spiritual support, and promote the patient's autonomy and dignity throughout their illness (Jeffrey, 2003). The NCHSPCS (1997) identified three levels of skills required to facilitate appropriate psychosocial support:

- **Level one:** General communication skills desirable for all carers.
- **Level two:** Skills including excellent interpersonal and communication skills appropriate to staff members with an extensive first-line role in palliative care (eg. clinical nurse specialists in palliative care).
- **Level three:** Skills that are required by an expert in psychosocial care (such as family therapist, chaplains and spiritual advisers, social workers, psychologists and psychiatrists).

(NCHSPCS, 1997; cited in Lloyd-Williams, 2003: 184)

Subsequently, many people receiving palliative care have their psychosocial support needs met by a range of professionals who have a variety of support skills (NCHSPCS, 1997). A significant number of palliative care patients may have complex psychological needs, which may require specialist intervention.

Psychosocial support for people with learning disabilities

Providing psychosocial support may be difficult for people with learning disabilities who are receiving palliative care in particular because of:

- The complexity of the learning disability itself (and often other associated disabilities) that might affect cognition and their understanding of their condition and its potential implications.
- Difficulties in reciprocal communication.
- Limited verbal communication skills.
- Limited ability to understand difficult concepts (such as treatment options and subsequent consequences, counselling and death).
- Difficulties in expressing feelings in socially acceptable and meaningful ways.
- Difficulties in recognising and articulating pain, distress and other associated symptoms.
- Having an external locus of control (which makes individuals totally reliant on others for their emotional support needs, eg. referral for specialist help).
- A history of disempowerment (emotional, philosophical and actual).
- Limited existing coping strategies and resources for the individual to draw upon.
- Disenfranchised grief and death (resulting in minimal exposure to the sad business of death and dying).
- A limited number of practitioners trained to work therapeutically with this population in the palliative care context.
- Limited resources from which to draw.
- Limited empirical research that supports such approaches (lack of evidence-based practice).

Additionally, the stigma often associated with disability, and the lack of knowledge about disabling conditions, might affect some professional carers' attitudes and responses. Such attitudes may lead to the emotional needs of people with learning disability being overlooked or ignored at a crucial time of their lives (ie. when faced with their own pending mortality) and often affect the accessibility of the usual emotional support networks (eg. counselling). Positive attitudes are an important feature of any care and support offered to people with learning disabilities, as Hollins (2003: viii) describes: 'The major barrier in the way of competent counselling provision for people with learning disabilities is not the presence of a learning disability, but the lack of understanding of the relevance of counselling by potential referrers'. Counselling is gradually emerging as a useful approach when working with people with a learning disability, but more empirical work is needed regarding its therapeutic effectiveness and the skills of the counsellor involved.

Counselling as helping

Within the literature, the need for a variety of psychotherapeutic approaches has been suggested when working with people with learning disabilities from differing therapeutic contexts, including individual (Cathcart, 1995; Kauffman, 1994) and group support (Rothenberg, 1994; French and Kuczaj, 1992; Read *et al*, 2001). From a bereavement perspective, more specialist interventions have been suggested which include guided mourning (Kitching, 1987; McEnhill, 1999), laughter therapy (Santiago-Cruz, 1999), psychotherapeutic support (Summers and Witts, 2003) and bereavement counselling (Read *et al*, 1999; Elliot, 1995; Read, 2001). Counselling is often perceived as one of a spectrum of helping activities (which include advice-giving, teaching, advocacy and information-sharing), delivered by a range of different professional groups from within a variety of differing care contexts. The characteristics of a helping relationship are described in *Panel 8.1*. They incorporate the qualities of empathy, congruency and unconditional positive regard — more commonly known as the core conditions (Rogers, 1957). Such qualities or conditions are frequently seen as crucial to any therapeutic relationship.

The British Association for Counselling (1984) defines counselling as 'work with individuals and with relationships which may be developmental, crisis support, psychotherapeutic, guiding or problem solving… The task of counselling is to give the "client" an opportunity to explore, discover and clarify ways of living more satisfying and resourcefully'. Counselling has also been more simply described as 'any situation in which the focus of a relationship is that one person is attempting to help another' (Parkes, Relf and Couldrick, 1996: 49), using a range of purposeful communication skills. However, Hodges (2003: 55) reminds us that 'counselling is not just about language and words, but about understanding' and, as such, may be difficult to access for people with learning disabilities (Conboy-Hill, 1992).

Accessing counselling as support

According to Parkes *et al* (1996), the majority of patients and families involved in palliative care do not seek formal counselling, but talk to those professionals involved in their continuing care; hence, counselling takes place 'within the context of a relationship which is primarily focused on non-counselling activities' (Parkes *et al*, 1996: 50). This is even more likely to be the case when offering palliative care for people with learning disabilities, since familiar carers are more likely to be able to communicate more easily with the individuals involved and vice versa. Therefore,

---

Panel 8.1: Characteristics of a helping relationship (Murry and Huelskoetter, 1997)

- **Being respectful** — feeling and communicating an attitude of seeing the client as a unique human being filled with dignity, worth and strengths, regardless of outward appearance or behaviour; being able to work at communicating with and understanding the client.
- **Being genuine** — communicating spontaneously, yet tactfully, what is felt and thought, with proper timing and without disturbing the client, rather than using jargon, façade or rigid counsellor role behaviours.
- **Being attentive** — conveying an active listening approach to verbal and non-verbal messages and promoting a positive attitude to working with the person.
- **Being positive** — showing warmth, care, respect; being able to reinforce the client for what he or she does well.
- **Being strong** — maintaining a separate identity from the client; withstanding the testing.
- **Being secure** — permitting the client to remain separate and unique; respecting their needs and your own; feeling safe as the client moves emotionally close; feeling no need to exploit the person.
- **Being knowledgeable** — having an expertise based on study, experience and supervision.
- **Being sensitive** — being perceptive to feelings; avoiding threatening behaviour; responding to cultural values, customs and norms as they affect behaviour; using knowledge that is pertinent to the client's situation; being kind and gentle.
- **Being empathic** — looking at the client's world from his or her viewpoint; being open to his or her values, feelings, beliefs and verbal statements; stating your understanding of his or her verbal or non-verbal expression of feelings and experiences.
- **Being non-judgemental** — refraining from evaluating the client moralistically or telling the client what to do.
- **Being congruent** — being natural, relaxed, honest, trustworthy, dependable and demonstrating consistency in behaviour between verbal and non-verbal messages.
- **Being unambiguous** — avoiding contradictory messages.
- **Being creative** — viewing the client as a person in the process of becoming, not bound by the past, and viewing yourself in the process of becoming or maturing as well.

---

whilst many healthcare professionals may not be trained counsellors, or indeed operating as trained counsellors, they may use a range of counselling skills when offering psychosocial support. This may also raise ethical and moral dilemmas and tensions as patients share personal thoughts and feelings that may not 'sit easily' within the professional's role, responsibility and, ultimately, duty of care. Clinical supervision and peer support will remain an important aspect within this professional role.

Palliative care usually brings about enormous changes in the patient's (and family members') lives, as people often struggle to make sense of what the illness is doing to them and their family (Parkes *et al*, 1996). Frank (1991) vividly describes his need to talk about his illness as 'disease talk' and 'illness talk':

> *Illness is the experience of living through the disease. If disease talk measures the body, illness talk tells of the fear and frustration of being inside a body that is breaking down. Illness begins where medicine leaves off... What happens to my body happens to my life.*

My life consists of temperature and circulation, but also of hopes and disappointments, joys and sorrows, none of which can be measured. Disease talk charts the progress of certain measures. Illness talk is a story about moving from a perfectly comfortable body to one that forces me to ask: what is happening to me?

Frank (1991: 13) cited in Parkes *et al* (1996: 50)

Talking about the illness, and sharing its impact and consequences with the patient and the family, may help both the person with the learning disability and family members to understand what is happening, whilst also affirming and clarifying the reality of the situation. Such openness may also encourage individuals to talk about their fears and aspirations, and to express their thoughts and feelings freely and safely. People with learning disability are described as being vulnerable within the death and dying situation (Read and Elliot, 2003), and invitations to talk and explore their illness and its effects may help to empower them and reduce this vulnerability.

A range of professionals may be involved in delivering holistic palliative care and should have a variety of skills, depending on their role and function within the palliative care team (NCHSPCS, 1997). Interpersonal skills are fundamental to this support; they also represent a way of relating to another person (Burnard, 1999) and are the foundation of good assessment (Parkes *et al*, 1996) and communication generally. They include skills such as active listening, exploring, clarifying and responding (Parkes *et al*, 1996). Professionals unfamiliar with people with a learning disability may have difficulties engaging with them in a meaningful way (for example, they may not be familiar with alternative communication systems) and familiar carers may have a pivotal role in aiding this communication process. Traditional methods of using dialogue as the main communication channel may have to be supplemented by other, more concrete methods, to promote more meaningful, reciprocal understanding. The pace of the communication may also be slower, as information and issues have to be repeated or language simplified for the purpose of understanding.

Person-centred approaches

Person-centred approaches to counselling (Rogers, 1957), including the core conditions of counselling — empathy, congruency and unconditional positive regard — have 'much to offer, both philosophically and clinically, for those who work with clients with mental retardation [*sic*]' (Prout and Cale, 1994: 116). 'Being empathic means having a "togetherness" with the client and, as a consequence, creating a trusting environment in which s/he feels cared for and safe' (Geldard 1998: 8). Metaphorically, empathy involves travelling as a companion alongside the client in his or her journey, seeing the world through their eyes, viewing the scenery along the way as they see it. Sympathy can be simplistically described as sitting across from someone and conveying how sorry or sad a person is about their situation; empathy, on the other hand, may be described as sitting next to the person and looking along the same path as is he or she, in an effort to understand and appreciate individual feelings and emotions. For some people with a learning disability, this may be a totally new experience as the counsellor seeks to understand their world and their views of it.

Congruency has been described by Machin (1998: 67) as 'a quality of transparency which permits a depth of engagement between counsellor and client' and, as such, is an important aspect of the counselling relationship. Such a relationship is established on trust, openness and understanding. Congruency involves being open, honest and genuine. Outside counselling, the counsellor assumes many roles as he or she seeks to balance personal and professional lives. The counsellor might also be a parent, a partner, a daughter, the captain of the local cricket club, or treasurer of the local darts team! During counselling, however, the counsellor does not assume any of these roles, as this would not be appropriate; but the experiences and skills involved in these other roles are part of what makes up the individual counsellor and makes them who they are.

When engaged in counselling, the counsellor may choose to disregard some of the other roles and associated skills and focus on those counselling and communication skills that will help to forge a working, reciprocal relationship. But what the counsellor brings to that relationship cannot easily be disengaged from what occurs outside the counselling arena. The counselling relationship involves a part of the counsellor and who they truly are — a genuineness and congruency — and the counsellor needs to recognise this.

Unconditional positive regard involves the total acceptance of the client with all their differences, strengths and weaknesses, in a non-judgemental way. 'Trust in the counsellor will deepen as acceptance and a condition of unconditional positive regard. However it does mean that "I accept the client as he is now, value him as a person, am non-judgemental of his behaviour and do not try to put my values upon him"' (Geldard, 1998: 8).

Such core conditions fundamentally underpin person-centred approaches to counselling, and researchers (eg. Machin, 1998) have subsequently identified a whole range of other indicative counselling principles and skills that need to be considered when offering counselling as support. Such principles and skills include safety, timing, confidentiality, listening with intent, reflection and clarification.

Person-centred approaches and people with learning disability

Prout and Strohmer (1994: 7) suggest that 'the less articulate client may feel uncomfortable in verbally orientated sessions'. Consequently, because of the complexities often involved in working with people with learning disabilities, counsellors (or those using counselling skills) may need to take a more directional role in focusing the content of any sessions. This may involve taking a more active conversational style of exchange between counsellor and client and involve more activities, such as role play, art work and life-story work (Prout and Strohmer, 1994).

Using person-centred approaches, the counsellor is essentially viewed as a facilitator to encourage the client's affective expression. Prout and Cale (1994) give an excellent account of the issues inherent in using person-centred approaches with this client group. Such issues encompass:

- The emphasis of worth and value and unconditional positive regard have an impact on both the counsellor and client behaviour. Positive attitudes and personal belief-systems are identified as being a crucial element in working with this client group and 'clearly the more positive regard we have for our clients with mental retardation [*sic*], the greater our efforts in working with them'.
- Many people with a learning disability are not used to people taking an active, unconditional interest in them. The many professionals involved in their lives are usually paid to be involved and are there for a variety of motives and reasons, overt and covert, frequently involving superior-inferior power relations.

- Many people with a learning disability may be compliant. Many do not dare refuse things (for example, contact with a bereavement counsellor) and, because of a history of suppression, may be reluctant or afraid (initially) to share or express their feelings.
- People with a learning disability may frequently be talked *at* as opposed to being talked *to* and may need time to adjust to this 'new' kind of relationship with 'trust and relationship-building' being of prime, initial concern.
- The counselling techniques used with people with a learning disability will be very similar to those used with non-disabled clients, but adaptations may be necessary to accommodate communication and language challenges: 'The counsellor may find it necessary to be somewhat more directive initially in order to get the client with mental retardation focused and expressing content relevant to pertinent issues'.

Prout and Cale (1994: 115–17)

This final comment about counsellors having to be more directive is an important aspect to consider within the counsellor's approach when working with this client group. Many people who have a learning disability have led such sheltered, protected and often suppressed lives that they often do not know what to ask for or what to do or explore to ease their sadness. The counsellor may have to help to empower the client to understand and appreciate the choices available to him or her by presenting options for consideration in a simple, concrete manner. Thus, the counselling may incorporate an educative function. Hurley (1989) presented a useful literature review around individual psychotherapy for people with learning disabilities and identified recommendations regarding guidelines for adapting effective therapeutic methods. These included:

- matching techniques to cognitive and developmental level
- using a directive approach
- remaining flexible in conducting therapy
- involving family and staff in the therapeutic process
- carefully managing transference and counter-transference issues
- addressing the disability as a specific issue.

Hurley (1989)

Such recommendations may be useful for anyone constructing guidelines in support of counselling or psychotherapy with this particular population in any counselling context.

In a small-scale study (Hawkins, 2002; n=8) to explore the experiences of counsellors using client-centred approaches with people with learning disabilities, counsellors were asked to identify the difficulties and dilemmas experienced when working with this population. Such difficulties incorporated both practical and philosophical issues and included: patience (due to the limited ability of the client to focus for long periods of time and becoming easily distracted); confidentiality (ie. maintaining boundaries within organisations); the negative attitudes of others about the value of counselling; accessing an appropriate venue (which affirms the value and worth of the counselling); a lack of social awareness of the clients involved; resources (staffing and transport that allows clients to continue with counselling); when the counselling philosophy and practice is not congruent with the general care environment's philosophy; disempowerment; trust; and general tiredness (Hawkins, 2002: 187–9). Such difficulties may affect how and where the counselling is conducted and the focus of the skills used.

During this study, counsellors were also asked to identify the particular rewards of working with this population (Hawkins, 2002). Such rewards included: the clients' emotional awareness and open, trusting nature; the small changes they saw as a result of their work; 'helping the most disempowered young people to experience themselves in a positive way'; a 'growth of their self-esteem and capacity to invite ideas and especially humour'; the 'simplicity and directness' that created engaging opportunities; and finding appropriate ways to meet (Hawkins, 2002; 189–90). These are rewards that any counsellor would aim for with any client population.

Since some people with learning disabilities may lack the emotional vocabulary to express their grief conventionally (Conboy-Hill, 1992) or discuss feelings about their illness or pending death, carers need to be creative in their approaches (French and Kuczaj, 1992). They need to use a range of media to promote understanding and nurture active engagement in a sensitive way. Such media may include diaries and photographs (Kennedy, 1989), which, in the palliative care context, can be used to record feelings, hopes and aspirations. Such activities may be useful in exploring a person's 'wish list' of outstanding achievements (such as going on holiday or visiting friends) to be fulfilled in the limited time available. Pictorial booklets (eg. Hollins, Dowling and Blackman, 2003) and the three booklets written by Cathcart (1994a, 1994b, 1994c) help inform individuals, families and professional carers about death, dying and bereavement issues. Activities such as the feelings or faces exercises (Heegaard, 1991) can help individuals recognise and explore their feelings in a simple and concrete manner. Read (1999) offers an introduction to such therapeutic approaches from a bereavement-counselling perspective, specifically in relation to people with learning disabilities. Many of these approaches (artwork, life-story and memory work, poetry, photographs and reminiscence work) can be usefully translated into working therapeutically with people with learning disabilities in a range of different contexts, including palliative care.

Promoting counselling and support

According to Parkes *et al* (1996: 70), professionals can promote counselling in palliative care generally by:

- Creating an environment in which it feels safe to express uncomfortable feelings, such as anger, guilt and sadness.
- Being non-judgemental and accepting of patients and their families.
- Being honest about what we know, or do not know, about the progression of the illness and being prepared to find out.
- Sharing our sadness about what is happening, or has happened, is awful, confusing and at times intolerable.

In addition to the factors above, when the person has a learning disability, professionals can also promote counselling in palliative care by:

- Treating individuals with adult status, and all that this entails.
- Involving the individual (as much as the person wants to be) in their care, treatment and options.

- Being prepared to use other non-verbal approaches to supplement verbal support (eg. audiotapes, books, photographs).
- Actively listen to individuals so that we have a clearer understanding of their needs and wants.
- Respecting their right to be involved in their care.
- Allowing extra time to explain, clarify or inform, using alternative, simpler language if necessary.
- Keeping ideas simple and concrete.
- Teaching an emotional vocabulary.
- Looking out for changes that might indicate distress.
- Being prepared to refer the person for specialist help.

Proactive approaches

The need for proactive educational opportunities to prepare people with learning disabilities for death and bereavement experiences has been identified by Yanok and Beifus (1993). They recommended community-based, instructional educational programmes (including visits to churches and cemeteries); instruction of standards of conduct for funerals; and proactive assistance to understand the broader contexts. On a practical note, they also recommended the use of simple language and avoidance of euphemisms surrounding death and a programme of continual development over months, rather than a concentrated effort over several days.

Group work has also been identified as a useful vehicle from which to explore sensitive issues around loss and change in an adult and meaningful way (Read *et al*, 2001; Read and Papakosta-Harvey, 2004; Read and Papakosta-Harvey, 2004). Group work can be used to explore, affirm and clarify perceptions of illness with this client population (before illness occurs) as part of a proactive educative programme. Many people with learning disabilities do have stories and experiences to share; given the right 'space' (ie. an open, honest, affirming, supportive, welcoming and nurturing approach) with a skilled facilitator, they may be willing to share these stories and experiences and learn from each other in an adult and human way.

Health promotion remains an important factor. Books such as *Keeping Healthy 'Down Below'* (Hollins and Downer, 2000) can be used from an educational perspective to encourage people with learning disabilities to consider and appreciate the importance of knowing one's own body and identifying changes, big or small. Exploring other people's experiences of serious illness and the treatment involved by using books (eg. *Getting on with Cancer*, Donaghey *et al*, 2002) might also improve individual understanding of the cancer journeys of others. Such resources have to be introduced sensitively and used in an informed and supportive environment.

Conclusion

This chapter has introduced the concept of psychosocial support in palliative care, particularly in relation to people with learning disabilities. It has explored counselling as part of the continuum of support and the challenges of offering counselling to people with learning disabilities. Counselling within the palliative care context is often sought from those carers directly involved in delivering palliative care who may not be trained counsellors. Therefore, those involved in providing palliative care should have effective interpersonal skills in order to address the emotional needs of their patients.

Accessing counselling for people with learning disabilities may be difficult for a range of philosophical and practical reasons; and in the palliative care context, time is a crucial element. People with a learning disability are more likely to seek emotional support from familiar carers, and the core conditions are identified as being important elements of this therapeutic relationship.

Research involving counselling and psychotherapeutic approaches is proportionately limited in relation to people with learning disabilities. More research is required to explore the nature of the emotional needs of people with learning disabilities who are dying. Although research with sensitive populations continues to be fraught with difficulties and challenges (ethically, morally, practically and scientifically), it is nonetheless imperative. Research that explores a range of therapeutic approaches and their effectiveness would ensure that appropriate emotional support is more readily available and enable the psychosocial needs of people with a learning disability who have a palliative illness to be met.

References

Badelt I (1990) Client-centred psychotherapy with mentally retarded adults. In: Lieter G, Rombauts J, Van Balen R (eds) (1990) *Client-Centred and Experiential Psychotherapy in the Nineties*. Leuven University Press, Leuven

British Association for Counselling (1984) *Code of Ethics and Practice for Counsellors*. BAC, Rugby

Burnard P (1999) *Acquiring Interpersonal Skills: a Handbook of Experiential Learning for Health Professionals*. 2nd edn. Stanley Thornes, Cheltenham

Cathcart F (1994a) *Understanding Death and Dying: Your Feelings*. British Institute of Learning Disabilities, Kidderminster, Worcs

Cathcart F (1994b) *Understanding Death and Dying: Your Feelings*. British Institute of Learning Disabilities, Kidderminster, Worcs

Cathcart F (1994c) *Understanding Death and Dying: Your Feelings*. British Institute of Learning Disabilities, Kidderminster, Worcs

Cathcart F (1995) Death and people with learning disabilities: interventions to support clients and carers. *Br J Clin Psychol* **34**: 165–75

Conboy-Hill S (1992) Grief, loss and people with learning disabilities. In: Waitman A, Conboy-Hill S (eds) (1992) *Psychotherapy and Mental Handicap*. Sage, London

Donaghey V, Bernat J, Tuffrey-Wijne I, Hollins S (2002) *Getting on with Cancer*. Gaskell/ St George's Hospital Medical School, London

Elliot D (1995) Helping people with learning disabilities to handle grief. *Nurs Times* **91**(43): 27–9

Frank AW (1991) At the will of the body: reflections on illness. In: Parkes CM, Relf M, Couldrick A (1996) *Counselling in Terminal Care and Bereavement.* BPS Books, Leicester

French J, Kucza J (1992) Working through loss and change with people with learning difficulties. *Ment Handicap* **20**: 108–11

Geldard D (1998) *Basic Personal Counselling: a Training Manual for Counsellors.* 3rd edn. Free Association Books, London

Hawkins J (2002) *Voices of the Voiceless: Person-Centred Approaches and People with Learning Difficulties.* PCCS Books, Ross-on-Wye

Heegaard M (1991) *When Mom and Dad Separate: Children Can Learn to Cope with Grief from Divorce.* Woodland Press, Minneapolis

Hewitt H, Branton P, Dunn J, Willcocks A (1997) Life story work: issues and applications for learning disabled people undergoing transition from hospital to community based settings. *J Learn Disabil Nurs Health Soc Care* **1**(3): 105–09

Hewitt H (2000) A life story approach for people with profound learning disabilities. *Br J Nurs* **9**(2): 90–5

Hodges S (2003) *Counselling Adults with Learning Disabilities.* Palgrave Macmillan, New York

Hollins S, Downer J (2000) *Keeping Healthy 'Down Below'.* Gaskell & St George's Hospital Medical School, London

Hollins S (2003) Foreword. In: Hodges S (2003) *Counselling Adults with Learning Disabilities.* Palgrave Macmillan, Hants

Hollins S, Dowling S, Blackman N (2003) *When Somebody Dies.* Gaskell & St.George's Hospital Medical School, London

Hurley AD (1989) Individual psychotherapy with mental retarded individuals: a review and call for research. *Res Dev Disabil* **10**: 261–75

James IA (1995) Helping people with learning disabilities to cope with bereavement. *Br J Learn Disabil* **23**: 74–8

Jeffrey D (2003) What do we mean by psychosocial care in palliative care? In: Lloyd-Williams M (ed) (2003) *Psychosocial Issues in Palliative Care.* Oxford University Press, Oxford

Kauffman J (1994) Mourning and mental retardation. *Death Studies* **18**: 257–71

Kennedy J (1989) Bereavement and the person with a mental handicap. *Nurs Stand* **1**(4): 36–8

Kitching N (1987) Helping people with mental handicaps cope with bereavement: a case study with discussion. *Ment Handicap* **15**: 61–3

Lloyd-Williams M (2003) *Psychosocial Issues in Palliative Care.* Oxford University Press, Oxford

Machin L (1998) *Looking at Loss: Bereavement Counselling Pack.* 2nd edn. Pavilion Publishing, Brighton

McDaniel B (1989) A group work experience with mentally retarded adults on the issues of death and dying. *J Gerontol Soc Work* **13**(3/4): 187–91

McEnhill L (1999) Guided mourning interventions. In: Blackman N (ed) (1999) *Living with Loss: Helping People with Learning Disabilities Cope with Bereavement and Loss*. Pavilion Publishing, Brighton

Murray RB, Huelskoetter MMM (1991) *Psychiatric/Mental Health Nursing: Giving Emotional Care*. 3rd edn. Appleton & Lange, Connecticut

National Council for Hospice and Specialist Palliative Care Services (1997) Feeling better: psychosocial care in specialist palliative care. London, Occasional Paper no. 13. In: Jeffrey D (2003) What do we mean by psychosocial care in palliative care? In: Lloyd-Williams M (cd) (2003) *Psychosocial Issues in Palliative Care*. Oxford University Press, Oxford

Parkes CM, Relf M, Couldrick A (1996) *Counselling in Terminal Care and Bereavement*. BPS Books, Leicester

Parkes CM (1998) The dying adult. In: Parkes CM and Markus A (eds) (1998) *Coping with Loss*. BMJ Books, London

Portner M (1990) Client-centred therapy with mentally retarded persons: Catherine and Ruth. In: Lieter G, Rombauts J, Van Balen R (eds) (1990) *Client-centred and Experiential Psychotherapy in the Nineties*. Leuven University Press, Leuven

Prout HT, Cale RL (1994) Individual counselling. In: Strohmer DC and Prout HT (eds) (1994) *Counselling and Psychotherapy with Persons with Mental Retardation and Borderline Intelligence*. Clinical Psychology Publishing Co, Vermont

Read S (1999) Creative ways of working when exploring the bereavement counselling process. In: Blackman N (ed) (1999) *Living with Loss: Helping People with Learning Disabilities Cope with Bereavement and Loss*. Pavilion Publishing, Brighton

Read S, Frost I, Messenger N, Oates S (1999) Bereavement counselling and support for people with a learning disability: identifying issues and exploring possibilities. *Br J Learn Disabil* **27**(2): 99–104

Read S, Papakosta-Harvey V (2004) Using workshops on loss for adults with learning disability: a second study. *J Learn Disabil* **8**(2): 191–208

Read S, Papakosta-Harvey V, Bower S (2001) Using workshops on loss for adults with learning disability. *Groupwork* **12**(2): 6–26

Read S (2001) A year in the life of a bereavement counselling service for people with learning disabilities. *J Learn Disabil* **5**(1): 19–33

Read S, Elliot D (2003) Death and learning disability: a vulnerability perspective. *J Adult Protect* **5**(1): 5–13

Rogers C (1957) The necessary and sufficient conditions of therapeutic personality change. *J Consul Psychol* **21**: 95–103

Rothenberg ED (1994) Bereavement intervention with vulnerable populations: a case report on group work with the developmentally disabled. *Soc Work Groups* **17**(3): 61–75

Santiago-Cruz R (1999) Pro-active approaches to loss and bereavement and maximising the quality of life of people with learning disabilities. Blackman N (ed) (1999) *Living with Loss: Helping People with Learning Disabilities Cope with Bereavement and Loss*. Pavilion Publishing, Brighton

Shirtliffe D (1995) Dramatic effect. *Nurs Times* **91**(21): 55–6

Summers SJ, Witts P (2003) Psychological interventions for people with learning disabilities who have experienced bereavement: a case study illustration. *Br J Learn Disabil* **31**: 37–41

Strohmer DC, Prout HT (eds) (1994) *Counselling and Psychotherapy with Persons with Mental Retardation and Borderline Intelligence*. Clinical Psychology Publishing Co, Vermont

Walker L, Walker M, Sharp D (2003) Current provision of psychosocial care within palliative care. Lloyd-Williams M (ed) (2003) *Psychosocial Issues in Palliative Care*. Oxford University Press, Oxford

Yanok J, Beifus JA (1993) Communicating about loss and mourning: death education for individuals with mental retardation. *Ment Retard* **31**(3): 144–7

CHAPTER 9

Spirituality, suffering and palliative care

John Swinton

I approached the writing of this chapter with some reservation. I have no doubt that people with learning disabilities have spiritual needs and that these needs are pertinent within a palliative care context (Swinton and Powrie, 2004; Raji, Hollins and Drinnan, 2003; James, 1995; McEvoy, Reid and Guerin, 2002). It is clear that people with learning disabilities in general want spirituality to be incorporated into the care and support that they receive (Swinton and Powrie, 2004; Swinton, 2002). When it comes to issues of life and death, many people with learning disabilities are more than able to express themselves and to develop constructive and informed responses to death, grief and loss (Swinton and Powrie, 2004; McEvoy *et al*, 2002). Spirituality is a significant presence in people's lives and, by extension, will be a significant presence in the way they die too. And yet, there is something about writing a chapter on 'the spiritual needs of people with learning disabilities' that makes me a little uncomfortable. The simple fact is that the spiritual and palliative needs of people with learning disabilities are the same as anyone else's. People with learning disabilities are people first and they share the same needs, hopes, desires, fears and expectations that all people do. Why then would one choose to single out this group of people and write a chapter on their 'special needs?' I don't think I have a satisfactory answer to this question.

It is fair to say that the palliative care of people with learning disabilities is a significantly under-researched area (Tuffrey-Wijne, 2002). Very little reflection has gone into exploring whether or not there are in fact any unique experiences or needs that people with learning disabilities encounter when faced with the process of dying. This is particularly so with regard to the spiritual dimensions of the experience of dying, which have received even less attention. So perhaps my justification for writing this chapter is that in attempting to offer some insights and clarity about the significance of the spiritual dimension for the palliative care of people with learning disabilities, I can at least raise people's consciousness to the importance of a dimension of palliative care that is often spoken about as important, but frequently omitted from the actual practice of care.

I therefore approach this chapter with caution. It is vital that readers recognise that the understanding of and insights into spirituality and spiritual care that I offer here are not for 'people with learning disabilities'; rather, they are relevant to all people, including those whom we choose to label 'learning disabled'. With these qualifying thoughts in mind, we can begin to reflect on the significance of spirituality for the palliative care of people with learning disabilities.

Developing an understanding of spirituality

A helpful place to begin our reflection is by trying to develop an initial understanding of 'spirituality'. Spirituality is a slippery concept that is not easily tied down. Trying to define spirituality is a little like trying to define love: you know what it is like when you feel it, but trying to capture it in words and concepts is tricky. The best you can do is indicate something of your experience and encourage others to recognise and discover the meaning of similar experiences within their own lives. In one sense, spirituality does not have a single meaning. It relates to an area of human experience that is filled with personal meaning and is, to an extent, unique to particular individuals. Diversity is almost inevitable. *Panel 9.1* summarises some of the ways in which the meaning of spirituality has been identified in the literature.

These definitions show the diverse ways in which spirituality is understood and defined and the variety of meanings that are ascribed to it. This diversity emerges from the uniqueness and individuality of spiritual experience and our struggle to find a conceptual language that can adequately capture its complex nuances.

Such diversity does not invalidate the clinical significance of spirituality. As David Hay (2002: 4) puts it, 'Like all interesting and important words, "spiritual" and "spirituality" have many shades of meaning'. The diversity does mean, however, that we will have to loosen our conceptual boundaries a little and become open to the importance of intuitive, experiential knowledge and

---

Panel 9.1: Descriptions of spirituality

- A sacred journey (Mische, 1982).
- The experience of the radical truth of things (Legere, 1984) and ultimate values (Cawley, 1997).
- Giving meaning and purpose in life (Legere, 1984; Clark et al, 1991; Fitchett, 1995; Sherwood, 2000).
- Relating to unconditional love (Ellison, 1983; Clark et al, 1991).
- Connectedness within oneself (Reed, 1992) and others (Sherwood, 2000).
- A life relationship or a sense of connection with mystery, a higher power, god or universe (Reed, 1992).
- A belief that relates a person to the world (Soeken and Carson, 1987).
- A quality that invokes a need to transcend the self in such a way that empowers, not devalues, the individual (Sherwood, 2000).
- Inner-dimension of being human attuned to the most valuable aspect of life that motivates and guides one's significant choices (Emblen, 1992).
- Being rooted in an awareness that is part of the biological make-up of the human species (Narayanasamy, 1999).
- Referring to meaning and unity, and a transcendent, usually referred to as 'God' in the West (Aldridge, 2000).
- That which gives meaning, purpose, hope and value to people's lives. This is part of a wide concept that may include, but is not defined by, religious faith and culture (Swinton, 2002).

From Narayanasamy, 2004. Reprinted here with permission of the author.

---

its significance for palliative care. As we reflect on the descriptions of spirituality offered above, we find that instead of hard conceptual definitions, we encounter a variety of themes that emerge from the human experience of 'the spiritual'. These themes, when taken seriously, can guide us into crucial and often hidden dimensions of patients' experiences that are often overlooked by the narrowness of our clinical gaze.

Understanding spirituality

We might pull together the descriptions presented above to say:

Spirituality is that dimension of a person's experience that relates to the search for meaning, purpose, hope and value, and opens up the possibility of connection with one another and with that which transcends ourselves.

A person's spirituality contains the beliefs, values, hopes and expectations that shape the structures of meaning that people use to interpret and make sense of their experiences, including their illness experiences. Within the context of palliative care, the way a person experiences their illness will, to a greater or lesser extent, depend on the way he or she sees and understands the world. These personal structures of meaning or significance give people a framework for understanding life-events and for making sense of experiences such as suffering and dying. Put simply, a person's spirituality relates to understanding and searching for an answer to the following questions:

- Who am I, where did I come to, where am I going and why?
- Who are you, where did you come from, where are you going to and why?
- Who are we? Where did we come from? Where are we going to and why?

Cotterell (1990)

Questions such as these become particularly poignant when a person becomes terminally ill. For some these questions will be answered through the spirituality of religion. Religions provide particular narratives, symbols, understandings and world-views that enable people to make sense of who they are in the world, why they have a particular illness, and how they should respond in the face of it. As such, religion can provide a vital resource for terminally ill patients who are trying to make sense of their illness experience.

Others will work out their quest for hope, meaning and love in other ways without any necessary reference to religion — for example, through meaningful relationships, art, nature and even employment.

The issue of the spirituality of employment is interesting. We live in a society that tends to base its systems of value on such things as competitiveness, power and employment. A person's job can often fulfill a spiritual role in their lives inasmuch as it provides meaning, purpose, value, identity and a sense of hope for the future. Thus, employment can be a primary way in which answers to fundamental questions are worked out.

A person's spirituality is thus seen to be unique, personal and can only truly be understood as carers relate meaningfully to the individual before them and begin to learn what spirituality means within the particular context of their lives. Even within religious traditions and the spirituality that emerges from them, there is a good deal of diversity of meaning and beliefs (Lartey, 2003; Augsberger, 1986). It is not possible to gauge what a person's spirituality means to them simply by looking at their label (eg. Christian, Jew, Buddhist, Humanist, Muslim). What is required is an understanding of the personal meanings of the individual's spirituality. We cannot assume anything about a person's spirituality without first entering into a meaningful relationship with them and beginning to understand how their spirituality is functioning within their unique illness experience. *Panel 9.2* provides an overview of spiritual needs in both their religious and non-religious forms.

What is palliative care?

Having laid down a foundational understanding of spirituality, it is necessary now to move on and explore in more detail precisely what we mean by the term 'palliative care'. The World Health Organisation (WHO) (2003) defines it thus (my bold):

> *Palliative care is an approach that **improves the quality of the life of patients** and their families facing the problems associated with life-threatening illness, through the **prevention and relief of suffering** by means of early identification and impeccable assessment and **treatment of pain and other problems physical, psychosocial and spiritual**.*
>
> WHO (2003)

Panel 9.2: An overview of spiritual needs in religious and non-religious forms

It is possible to divide spiritual needs into six main categories (Emblem and Holstead, 1993):

- **Religious needs**
  Facilitation of discussions about the transcendent aspects of human existence
  Prayer
  Scripture reading
  Confession/catharsis
  Forgiveness

- **Values/structures of meaning**
  Hope
  Faith
  Search for meaning/purpose to life
  Dealing with guilt

- **Relationships**
  The need for human presence
  The possibility of intimacy

- **Transcendence**
  Dimensions other than physical/mental
  Assurance of God's presence
  Inner-need—inner-person

- **Affective feeling**
  Reassurance
  Comfort
  Peace
  Happiness

- **Communication**
  Talking
  Listening and being listened to

From Swinton (1999a).

The WHO's definition enables us to understand palliative care in terms of three primary functions:

1. Relieving suffering.
2. Improving quality of life.
3. Enabling individuals and families to experience a good death.

For current purposes, I will focus primarily on the first of these functions, which, in effect, underpins and determines the other two: the relief of suffering. I will suggest that it is in the prevention and relief of suffering that spirituality finds a primarily role in palliative care. Reflecting on the nature of suffering will help show the importance of the spiritual dimension for palliative care.

Suffering and palliative care

The most obvious source of suffering for people living with terminal illness is of course pain. The connection of pain and suffering is so natural that we rarely think beyond it. Quite rightly so; pain is a significant source of suffering and one that most of us naturally try to avoid. However, pain is only one (and not always the most important) dimension of suffering. Eric Cassell (1982: 640) argues that suffering occurs when:

> *an impending destruction of the person is perceived; it continues until the threat of disintegration has passed or until the integrity of the person can be restored in some other manner. It follows, then, that although suffering often occurs in the presence of acute pain, shortness of breath, or other bodily symptoms, suffering extends beyond the physical. Most generally, suffering can be defined as a state of severe distress associated with events that threaten the intactness of the person.*

Cassell points out that suffering is not confined to physical symptoms; is not measurable in terms of pain alone; and it cannot be assessed on a scale that is universal (ie. applicable to all people irrespective of context, personality and situation). Rather, suffering occurs when a person experiences a loss of meaning, purpose, hope and value, which leads to a form of disintegration of the self. Suffering is unique to individuals and filled with personal meaning. As McCurdy (2002) puts it:

> *suffering is personal, it has to do with the meanings that illness (and treatment) hold for this person. Ultimately, a key ingredient of suffering is the person's experience of a threat to integrity or 'intactness' — in any or all dimensions of life, the bodily among them.*

McCurdy (2002) goes on to suggest that 'the meaning that illness or injury holds for a person depends on factors in that person's history and relationships that others simply do not know'. Suffering is a deeply personal thing that relates to the person's personality, their unique life experiences, their expectations, values, hopes and the particular ways in which they see and understand the world. What Cassell and McCurdy point towards is the fact that the degree of suffering a person will experience is closely tied in with the meaning that is placed on the event that causes the suffering and the consequences of the interpretation of their situation and themselves within it. Suffering of this type is inherently spiritual.

Importantly, both writers point to the connection between suffering and a person's experience of impending destruction and disintegration. Within a palliative care context, the idea of impending destruction and disintegration appear relatively straightforward insofar as the particular terminal illness the patient is encountering will bring these things about in a physical sense. However, in practice, the destruction and disintegration is more than simply physical death: it relates to other dimensions of a person's experience, such as the destruction of meaning and hopes for the future; the destruction of a sense of value and purpose; the desolation of self-image and identity caused by disfiguring diseases or treatments; the disintegration of faith in the face of impending death; the destruction (both real or anticipated) of relationships in response to bereavement and loss; the separation of a person from God through the shattering of faith, which can accompany diagnosis; and the destruction of the social self brought on by the social alienation and stigma that accompanies certain terminal illnesses, such as AIDS and cancer (Sontag, 2001).

People with learning disabilities can be particularly prone to such forms of suffering. There is a good deal of literature that suggests that people with learning disabilities are a devalued population who struggle to find sources of value and acceptance within a society that is prone to stigmatising and alienating that which is perceived to be different (Curtice, 2001; Swinton, 1999b; Vanier, 1992). This social devaluation has important implications for the quality of their lives, their ability to attain acceptance and meaningful citizenship — and their experience of palliative care. Claude Regnard (2003) has highlighted the significance of 'diagnostic overshadowing', which he describes as:

The inability to see possible ill-health and conditions that may be present beyond the learning disability.

(SHS Trust, 2003: 18)

Learning disability is a 'totalising label'. In other words, when a person is given the label 'learning disabled', it doesn't simply apply to one aspect of a person: it is generalised as a way of understanding everything that the person does and experiences, including the way they experience illness. What Regnard highlights is the danger of carers assuming that particular experiences and desires are not present because of the learning disability. The label 'learning disability' thus blocks the suffering from the eyes of carers who can only see what they assume they will see according to their understanding of the term 'learning disabled'. When this happens, the severity of the person's suffering is underestimated or overlooked completely; they are then left to face their suffering alone. Within a palliative care context, this can lead to forms of care that are strong on pain control and functional care, but significantly lacking in emotional and spiritual dimensions.

The process of diagnostic overshadowing is not necessarily conscious. It can often be a product of the negative ways in which we are socialised into viewing people with learning disabilities. Linda McEnhill, drawing on the ideas of Valerie Sinason, a psychologist working at the Tavistock Institute in London, suggests that people with learning disabilities live in a 'death-making culture' (Sinason's phrase; Sinason, 1996; McEnhill, 2003). Within a death-making culture 'the messages sent out by the media in many cases imply that it is a tragedy for a person with a learning disability to be born' (McEnhill, 2003). Within such a culture, older mothers are encouraged to take tests to see if their children are disabled and to think about terminations if the answer is positive. Births of learning-disabled children are not celebrated. Within this death-making culture, many people with learning disabilities grow up with a strong negative message, something like: 'People like me shouldn't exist; I shouldn't exist; my parents' lives would be better without me' (McEnhill, 2003). McEnhill suggests that these negative messages, which begin at birth, often affect the context in which a person with a learning disability faces terminal illness. This has three important implications:

1. It can stop people taking action to prevent disease.
2. It can stop people thinking they have a right to prolonged life.
3. It can create a culture where some people with disabilities and carers may secretly believe that life is not valued and death is a blessing (McEnhill, 2003).

There can be a tendency to await the person's death rather than celebrate the quality of his or her life. When this happens, death can only be thought of negatively as a relief, a blessing, or even a 'good thing' in that it enables families to be happy again. It is clear then that diagnostic overshadowing is an important potential cause of suffering and has significant interpersonal and social dimensions that are vital for a spiritually informed holistic understanding of palliative care. While most of what has been said in this chapter could be applied to all people, this dimension of the suffering of people with learning disabilities presents a unique challenge for palliative carers.

Meaning and suffering

Whilst some of the suffering experienced by people with learning disabilities has social roots, there are also some vital personal and interpersonal dynamics that carers need to recognise. Central amongst these is 'meaning'. The process of dying evokes a crisis of meaning that can plunge people into personal crisis and evoke the type of disintegration of the self that has been discussed. Fife (1994: 309) describes meaning in the following way:

The concept of meaning commonly refers to the relationship between individuals and their world, as well as to individuals' unique perceptions of their place within that world. It is these perceptions that give a sense of coherence to life in the face of loss, change and personal upheaval. Meaning becomes particularly significant in the realm of stress and coping with serious illness because such an extraordinary event imposes irrevocable change that totally disrupts the continuity of everyday life. Consequently people are forced to re-define the meanings they have assumed, or supposed as fact in the routine of living.

Meaning is thus seen to be a personal thing that relates to the structures of significance that a person creates during their lifetime to enable them to make sense of their experience and retain a sense of coherence and wholeness in the midst of life's changes and uncertainties. Serious illness challenges our understandings of the way the world should be and threatens the structure of the way that we have created our personal, social universes. Because it challenges the way that we assume the world to be, the meanings we have developed in the world can begin to crumble as the resources we have accumulated to ensure the maintenance of meaning begin to let us down. In short, terminal illness brings a loss of meaning that can lead to intense suffering.

It is important to remember that meaning is unique to particular individuals. What is meaningful for one person will not necessarily be meaningful for another; what is important for one person may not be important for others; what is important at one moment in time may not be at another. So, for example, it may be that for a patient with a strong religious faith who discovers that she has a terminal illness, death is not the main problem. The religious structures through which she has developed ways of living in and making sense of the world may well offer her an understanding of death that is non-threatening, hopeful and comforting.

However, although the thought of death may not cause suffering in itself, other dimensions of the process of dying may do so. For example, suffering may be brought on by the thought of leaving loved ones behind. Whilst death in itself may be faced hopefully, the sense of disappointment at being separated from loved ones may be a source of great sadness and distress. Issues of broken relationships and reconciliation may emerge as sources of suffering. The process of dying often initiates a process of reflection wherein a person brings to mind various key points in their lives and begins to think them afresh. Broken relationships often re-emerge and need to be re-thought and perhaps reconciled. This can be problematic if the person with whom they want to be reconciled is no longer available. It can be even more problematic if the dying person has high communicational needs that make it difficult for those around her to recognise the locus of her suffering. In this type of situation, it is very easy to put the distress of a person with learning disabilities down simply to the physical process of dying and to overlook its spiritual and emotional dimensions.

The important thing is to search for the source of the crisis of meaning and to reflect with the person on how best to restore that meaning. So, for example, it has been suggested that a person's employment provides meaning, purpose and hope for their lives and offers them acceptance and inclusion, social status and a positive sense of value, identity and citizenship. To lose this source of spiritual fulfilment through illness can be as devastating as the illness itself. If a person is no longer able to manage to attend their place of work, this can present a huge gap in their structures of meaning and evoke a significant loss of self-identity leading to depression, anxiety, sadness, disconnection and uncertainty about who they are and why they are in the world. Similarly, if a person's primary social network is intricately connected to their workplace and that source of connection is no longer available, this can seriously exacerbate the sense of loneliness, alienation and disconnection that accompany the experience of terminal illness. Bearing in mind the significance of employment for many people with learning disabilities, this may well be an important dimension of suffering for some people.

The meaning of religious spirituality in relation to palliative care

If a person holds religious beliefs, these may well be positively used to cope with the experience of terminal illness. There is evidence to suggest that religion can be a powerful coping mechanism

(Pergament, 2001). Emerging research findings would suggest that this is so for people with learning disabilities too (Swinton and Powrie, 2004). A religious belief system provides people with specific ways of viewing and understanding the world. They offer people structures, concepts and language that individuals can use in their attempts to make sense of their illness experience. Such belief systems can be a source of hope, possibility and meaning in the face of apparent hopelessness and meaninglessness. As such, religion can be a powerful protective force against suffering.

However, the discovery of terminal illness can also bring about a profound crisis of faith. The process of dying may cause a person to question their own beliefs and lead to anxiety and uncertainty about the future (Sheldon, 1998; Byrne, 2002). The process of dying can separate people from self, others and their god. It can separate people from themselves in that they now discover they have a new identity which may be very different from the old one (eg. patient, dying person, ex-workmate, etc). Here, diagnostic overshadowing takes on another turn as people now find their identity subsumed by their diagnosis of terminal illness. This new identity means that all the hopes and possibilities the person had for the future have now gone (or at best been radically altered). The person is faced with a very different future. People find themselves dislocated from their old selves and struggle to find out who this new 'terminally ill' person is.

The process of dying also separates persons from others insofar as those around the person 'don't have what she has'; the person with a terminal illness is no longer 'like them' and if those around them don't want to talk about their concerns, fears and experiences, then this separation is deepened and a person's sense of alienation compounded. Bearing in mind the stigma, isolation and sense of being perceived as 'different' that mark the lives of many people with learning disabilities, to have this alienation compounded with a new label and a new form of exclusion in the midst of the pain and anxiety of terminal illness will inevitably exacerbate their suffering.

Terminal illness can also separate a person from their God because it disappoints them. Many religious traditions talk of a God who loves human beings, who wants what is best for them and, at times, who heals them. When this image is challenged by the experience of terminal illness, people experience deep suffering, anxiety and sometimes guilt. They might ask, 'Why is this happening to me?', 'What is it that I have done to deserve this?' and 'Why has my God allowed this to happen to me?' Thus, terminal illness can bring about a deep crisis of faith within religious patients. This may be expressed verbally for those who have this capacity, but it may also be expressed non-verbally through disturbed behaviour, withdrawal and anxiety.

It is clear, then, that spirituality and a deeper understanding of the nature of suffering are a crucial dimension of palliative care.

Spiritual care

In closing this chapter, I will highlight three basic dimensions within the process of the spiritually orientated palliative care of people with learning disabilities. If carers can grasp these three dimensions, then the process of spiritual care will have begun. As before, I stress that these dimensions are relevant for all people and not intended to be special or unique to the situation of people with learning disabilities.

1. Remembering the person

The care team must remember that the patient before them is first and foremost a person and that each person's illness takes place within a unique system of personal meanings and values that may be crucial in understanding and coping with terminal illness. The person may have a terminal illness, and they may carry the label of 'learning disabled', but it is their identity as unique persons that must remain primary. The subtle dynamics of diagnostic overshadowing can easily slip into the practice of palliative care when carers are faced with a person who is perceived to be 'different' and to have different needs from 'normal' people. It is very easy for all of us to fall into the trap of assuming that people with learning disabilities 'couldn't cope with discussions about sensitive topics', 'wouldn't understand death', 'can only have a child-like faith' or 'should be protected from talking about certain things *for their own good*'. It is clear from the literature that many people with learning disabilities have a firm grasp of issues surrounding death and its implications for their lives, and are able to discuss intimate and difficult topics surrounding death and dying (Swinton and Powrie, 2004; Read, 1996). To assume otherwise is depersonalising and may well reflect a discomfort on the part of carers to address certain issues, rather than an inability of the learning-disabled person to conceptualise and work through complex emotional and spiritual issues. In remembering that the person with a learning disability is first and foremost a person with unique understandings, beliefs, values, desires and hopes, the possibility of creating a context within which such experiences can be expressed, recognised and valued becomes a reality.

2. Suffering and personhood

We have seen that suffering occurs when the integrity of the person is threatened or disrupted. Such suffering continues until the threat has been removed or the integrity of the person restored. It is crucial to recognise that the intensity of a person's suffering can only be measured on the patient's terms. It is the level of distress that they feel they are experiencing and their assessment of the seriousness of the threat or problem that is paramount. People with learning disabilities, like most people in a palliative-care context, may struggle to understand the technical details of their condition. Indeed, the clinical details of their pathology may not matter to people. What does matter is how their condition affects their personal lives. It is therefore not enough simply to be aware of the technical details of a person's condition; to deal with their suffering, it is necessary to understand the unique, personal meanings of someone's life and to grasp the meanings of their goals, values, beliefs, hopes and expectations. Spiritual care begins when we recognise that 'patients' are unique persons and strive to enter into forms of relationship that will enable carers to access and understand the inner dynamics of the patient's suffering. Developing such understanding requires carers to ask difficult questions:

- What is most important for you just now?
- What is it that you are frightened of?
- What is it that makes you most sad about your situation?
- What do you worry is going to happen to you?

- What is the worst thing about all of this?
- What do you hope for?
- What will you miss most about the way that your life was before the illness?

Of course carers will have to be comfortable with dealing with the answers to these questions. It is clear from the wider literature that often they are not (Oldnall, 1996). There is clearly a need for education and training within the area of spirituality and spiritual care if people with learning disabilities (and indeed all people) are to receive effective spiritual care that dares to ask and to help the person answer questions such as these.

3. Recognising and understanding

It has been suggested that the process of dying brings about a crisis of meaning. If so, then in order to address spiritual needs, carers must seek to understand the unique meaning of the patient's experiences and stories within the context of their beliefs, family and cultural values (Association of American Medical Colleges; cited in Post *et al*, 2000). Facilitating spiritual care and the reconstruction of meaning requires carers to place themselves in a position where they can recognise, validate and help facilitate the feelings of the person to whom they are offering care. Spiritual carers must listen with at least three questions in mind:

- What is it that is giving meaning and hope to this person's life?
- In what way is the process of dying affecting these structures of meaning?
- How best can I/we facilitate a reconstruction of meaning that will enable this person to have a good death?

How these questions are answered depends of course on the particular needs of the individual. However, before any answers can be worked through, the carer needs to develop a degree of empathy that will enable her to be open to the possibility of this type of spiritual need and a willingness to enter into healing dialogue (verbal and non-verbal) that will recognise, respect and enable reconnection and new meaning. At a basic level, this might mean, for example, simply recognising that a person's relationship with his girlfriend may be the most significant dimension of his life, and making sure that she is able to visit him regularly. It might mean ensuring that any family tensions around the couple get the opportunity to be resolved, and that the girlfriend has the emotional support to allow her to cope with the process of losing her loved one. Here, spiritual care focuses on enabling access to that which gives the patient meaning, purpose and hope, and strives to create the circumstances in which that dimension of their lives can be nurtured and sustained. In this case, the locus of intervention is not the dying person, but their social network.

Again, if employment is highly significant for a person's sense of meaning and purpose, spiritual care might involve ensuring that work colleagues get the opportunity to visit regularly and that the dying person is able to retain their identity as part of the workforce team, even though participation in the workplace may be minimal or non-existent.

If a person has a religious faith, spiritual care may take the form of referral to the chaplain or a religious leader. If the carer has a shared religious faith, they may wish to pray with the patient or talk through the various concerns and hopes that inevitably emerge. Bearing in mind the significance of relationships for the spirituality of people with learning disabilities (Swinton, 2002), spiritual care may relate to reconnecting with friends from within the religious community and allowing them to accompany the person on their quest for meaning and their journey towards death. The important thing for all carers is to be aware of the nature of a person's spiritual needs and to be able and willing to explore them as and when they arise.

Spiritual care as journeying

These initial three dimensions of spiritual care mean that carers have to take an approach to care that is recognisably different from the way in which professionals often conceptualise their relationships to patients. The approach outlined thus far demands that we learn to journey with people with learning disabilities as they move towards death. 'Journeying' in its basic meaning is the act of travelling from one place to another; within the context of palliative care, this means travelling with the patient as she moves from her present life, with all of its hopes and expectations, towards death and all that that may mean for her. Journeying demands that we enter into meaningful, empathic relationships that enable us to understand and to be with the unique individual before us. It demands that we become fellow travellers who try to see the world the way our patients do, and to communicate a sense of solidarity as they encounter the various twists and turns of the dying process.

A focus on spiritual journeying demands that carers genuinely enter into the experience of the patient and try, as far as they can, to understand the real meaning of their experience and the implications of that meaning for the strategies of care that are adopted. This can be painful, complicated and deeply challenging, both personally and professionally. To enter into the experience of another is to open one's self up to the possibility of experiencing suffering and most of us do not court that with enthusiasm. Certainly, professional distance may be necessary in order that certain clinical judgements can be made and patients can be protected from unhealthy forms of involvement which might restrict rather than increase the quality of their lives. Nevertheless, journeying as an aspect of spiritual care does demand of us a different form of relationship, which will enable us genuinely and meaningfully to journey with the dying person and to help them deal with their suffering on their terms and in the ways that are most meaningful for them.

Conclusion

My intention in this chapter has not been to provide a systematic scheme to tell carers how to do spiritual care — this is not what is required. Spiritual care is not simply a series of actions that need to be carried out: it is a way of being with another person within which one opens up one's self to the possibility of recognising hidden dimensions of suffering and learns to respond in ways that are compassionate, empathic and sensitive to the importance of the person's spiritual quest. In other words, spiritual care is not something that should be understood apart from what we already do on a daily basis; it has to do with carrying out our daily tasks with a new sensitivity to the significance of spirituality and the subtleties of human suffering. Spiritual care relates to the care team learning to see the person before them differently — as a spiritual being with needs, hopes, values, beliefs and expectations that transcend the boundaries of technical thinking. It is about recognising these needs as integral to the process of palliative care and not as something 'added on' to the real task of caring. It is about seeing what we are already doing in a different light. When we begin to see people differently, our response to and understanding of their situation will inevitably change. This shift in our response and understanding is the beginning point of spiritual care.

Of course, there are certain things that carers need to learn: the nature of spirituality; the need for spiritual empathy; the nature of spiritual needs; the importance of meaning and relationships; the significance of religious traditions; when to refer; the role of the chaplain; and so forth. However, before we can effectively learn these types of skills, we need to begin with a change in the way we view the person before us; we need to develop an understanding of the person as a spiritual being whose experience of suffering and dying is unique, complex and absolutely crucial to the process of palliative care.

It is my hope that this chapter will at least begin to open carers' minds to the possibility that spirituality might be of relevance to the task of palliative care and move us all to begin to think seriously about the most effective ways in which we can explore this dimension with patients. Some might argue that they are already doing all of these things; if so, I am delighted. However, the literature would suggest that most professional carers are uncertain about the spiritual dimension to the extent that they exclude it from their professional practice (Oldnall, 1996). There remains much to be done in enabling effective palliative care that incorporates people's spiritual needs as a central dimension of care.

References

Aldridge D (2000) *Spirituality, Healing and Medicine*. Jessica Kingsley, London

Augsberger DW (1986) *Pastoral Counselling Across Cultures*. Westminster Press, Philadelphia

Bassett RL, Perry K, Repass R, Silver E, Welch T (1994) Perceptions of God among persons with mental retardation: a research note. *J Psychol Theol* **22**(1): 45–9

Byrne M (2002) Spirituality in palliative care: what language do we need? *Int J Palliat Nurs* **8**(2): 67–74

Cassell EJ (1982) The nature of suffering and the goals of medicine. *New Engl J Med* **306**(11): 639–45

Cawley N (1997) Toward defining spirituality: an exploration of the concept of spirituality. *Int J Palliat Nurs* **3**(1): 31–6

Clark CC, Cross JR, Deane DM, Lowery LW (1991) Spirituality: integral to quality care. *Holist Nurs Pract* **5**(3): 67–76

Cotterell P (1990) *Mission and Meaninglessness*. SPCK, London

Curtice L (2001) The social and spiritual inclusion of people with learning disabilities: a liberating challenge? *Contact Interdisciplin J Past Studies* **36**: 15–23

Ellison CW (1983) Spiritual well–being: conceptualization and measurement. *J Psychol Theol* **11**: 4

Emblen JD, Halstead L (1993) Spiritual needs and interventions: comparing the views of patients, nurses and chaplains. *Clin Nurse Spec* **3**(7): 175–82

Fife BL (1994) The conceptualization of meaning in illness. *Soc Sci Med* **38**: 309–14

Fitchett G (1995) Linda Krauss and the lap of God: a spiritual assessment case study. *Second Opin* **20**(4): 40–9

Hay D (2002) The spirituality of adults in Britain — recent research. *Scot J Health Chaplain* **4**: 6

James IA (1995) Helping people with learning disability to cope with bereavement. *Br J Learn Disabil* **23**(2): 74–8

Lartey EY (2003) *In Living Colour: an Intercultural Approach to Pastoral Care and Counselling*. Jessica Kingsley, London

Legere T (1984) A spirituality for today. *Studies in Formative Spirituality* **5**(3): 514–20

McCurdy D (2002) Medicine, religion and the experience of suffering. *Oates Journal* **5**: http://www.oates.org/journal/vol-05-2002/articles/abst-mccurdy-01.html

McEnhill (2003) Philosophical barriers: a death-making culture. In: *Palliative Care and People with Learning Disabilities* (2003). SHS Trust

McEvoy J, Reid Y, Guerin S (2002) Emotion recognition and concept of death in people with learning disabilities. *Br J Develop Disabil* **48**(95): 83–9 [part 2]

Mische P (1982) Toward a global spirituality. In: Mische P (ed) *The Whole Earth Papers*. Global Education Association, East Orange, New Jersey

Narayanasamy A (2004) Palliative Care and Spirituality. Unpublished paper used here with permission

Narayanasamy A (1999) A review of spirituality as applied to nursing. *Int J Nurs Stud* **36**: 117–25

Oldnall A (1996) A critical analysis of nursing: meeting the spiritual needs of patients. *J Adv Nurs* **23**: 138–44

Pargament KI (2001) *The Psychology of Religion and Coping: Theory, Research, Practice*. Guilford Press

Post SG (1995) *The Moral Challenge of Alzheimer Disease*. Johns Hopkins University Press, London

Raji O, Hollins S, Drinnan A (2003) How far are people with learning disabilities involved in funeral rites? *Br J Learn Disabil* **31**(1): 42–5

Regnard C (2003) *Palliative Care and People with Learning Disabilities*. SHS Trust

Read S (1996) Helping people with learning disabilities grieve. *Br J Nurs* **5**(2): 91–5

Reed P (1992) An emerging paradigm for the investigation of spirituality in nursing. *Res Nurs Health* **15**: 349–57

Sheldon F (1998) ABC of palliative care: bereavement. *BMJ* **316**: 456–8 (7 Feb)

Sherwood G D (2000) The power of nurse-client encounters. *J Holist Nurs* **18**(2): 159–75

SHS Trust (2003) Palliative Care and People With Learning Disabilities. http://www.ckglasgow. org.uk/pdf/pallcare_sep03.pdf

Soeken KL, Carson VJ (1987) Responding to the spiritual needs of the chronically ill. *Nurs Clin North Am* **22**(3): 603–11

Sontag S (2001) *Illness as Metaphor.* Picador, USA

Stiemke FA (1994) Church synagogue-temple-mosque advocacy: an avenue for integration in religious and secular communities. *J Rel Disabil Rehab* **1**(4): 1–11

Swinton J Powrie E (2004) Why are we here?: the spiritual lives of people with learning disabilities. The Foundation for People with Learning Disabilities, London

Swinton J (2002) A space to listen: meeting the spiritual needs of people with learning disabilities. The Foundation for People with Learning Disabilities, London

Swinton J (1999a) Reclaiming the soul: a spiritual perspective on forensic nursing. In: Robinson D, Kettles A (eds) *Forensic Nursing and Multidisciplinary Care of the Mentally Disordered Offender.* Jessica Kingsley, London

Swinton J (1999b) *Building a Church for Strangers: Theology, Church and Learning Disabilities.* Contact Pastoral Trust, Edinburgh

Tuffrey-Wijne I (1997) Palliative care and learning disabilities. *Nurs Times* **93**(31): 50–1

Tuffrey Wijne (2002) The palliative care needs of people with intellectual disabilities: a case study. *Int J Palliat Nurs* **8**(5): 222–32

Sinason V (1992) *Mental Handicap and the Human Condition: New Approaches from the Tavistock.* Free Association Books, London

Vanier J (1992) *From Brokenness to Community.* Paulist Press, New York

World Health Organisation (WHO) (2003) http://www.who.int/cancer/palliative/definition/en/

CHAPTER 10

The role of hospices

Linda S McEnhill

You matter because you are you and you matter until the last moment of your life. We will do all we can, not only to help you die peacefully but to live until you die.
Dame Cicely Saunders (1964)

The modern hospice movement dates back to 1967 when Dame Cicely Saunders opened St Christopher's Hospice in London. However, the word 'hospice' is much older, dating back to the fourth century when it was used to describe a place of rest. In its original usage, it would have denoted a stopping-off place for pilgrims, travellers or strangers, as well as a home for the destitute (*Shorter English Dictionary*, 1988).

The contemporary use of the word 'hospice', to denote care of the dying, began in 1842 when it was used by Mme Jeanne Garnier, who founded the Dames De Calvaire in Lyon, France. It was used again in this way in 1879 when the Irish Sisters of Charity opened Our Lady's Hospice in Dublin, Ireland, followed by St Joseph's Hospice in Hackney, London, in 1905, run by the same religious order (Hospice Information Service, 2003).

Today, hospices are no longer humble stopping-off places; indeed, many of them regard themselves as 'specialist palliative care units'. However, they have tried, despite the pressures of a constantly changing health culture, to maintain the idea that they are as much about hospitality as they are about symptom control.

One of the principle changes in the hospice model in its fairly short lifespan is the move away from building-based services to community-based services. Thus, although there are 222 inpatient units in the UK (2005), they are predominately resource centres that serve a much larger number of patients and families in the community than their combined 3,156 inpatient beds could ever hope to manage (Hospice Information Service, 2005). From these centres, Macmillan nurse and community palliative care teams operate. Increasingly, there is the development of 'hospice at home teams' bringing everything into the patient's home, which would previously have only been available within hospice buildings. This development has special relevance in trying to enable the 75% of people who say they wish to die at home to do so, as opposed to the 25% who are presently able to do so. The development of 263 day-hospice centres (either within bedded units or independently) has also made a significant contribution to the quality of life for both patients and families.

However, the hospice movement has grown in an uneven and, some would say, unfair manner, with some areas having good hospice provision and others having little or none. This is primarily related to the lack of statutory funding in its development. Of the 220 hospice inpatient units presently in the UK, only sixty-four are NHS-managed. The remaining 156 have developed as the result of the activity of national charities (Marie Curie with ten units and Sue Ryder with six) and by the good will and determination of local communities (140 units).

The children's hospice movement

The children's hospice movement is a latecomer to the scene with the first unit only being developed in 1983. It has grown fairly rapidly and there are now thirty-three children's hospices. Their funding situation, however, is even less favourable, with only a very small amount of their funding being derived from statutory sources.

Thus, although great things have been achieved by the hospice movement begun by Cicely Saunders, her dream that it would change the face of general care such that it would become obsolete has not yet been realised. It is still the case that, even with well-developed systems of palliative care delivered in a range of settings, the majority of statutory funding goes to fund 'curative' treatments (despite their woefully low success rates). Very little funding, comparatively, goes to the palliation of symptoms and care of those dying of thus far 'incurable' diseases.

Disadvantaged dying and the hospice movement

Whilst most people would consider the dying to be a 'disadvantaged group' in their own right, this term has been used to signify specific groups of dying individuals who are under-represented in accessing the full range of palliative-care services appropriate to them (DoH, 2003). Amongst these groups are prisoners, refugees and asylum seekers, as well as people suffering from mental-health conditions.

It is only recently that people with learning disabilities have been recognised as constituting another of the disadvantaged dying groups. It has been known for some time that people with learning disabilities are under-represented in primary healthcare services, despite their healthcare needs being significantly higher than the non-learning disabled population. A number of attempts have been made to address this through healthcare policy (DoH, 1995; DoH, 1998), most recently in the Government's White Paper *Valuing People* (DoH, 2001). However, little attention has been given to their needs when encountering terminal illness or bereavement. Some researchers, for example Todd (2002), offer suggestions, echoing earlier writing by authors such as Sinason, as to why this may be the case. The lack of care for people with learning disabilities is seen to be both a concrete expression of society's 'death wish' towards people with learning disabilities, and an effect of the infantalisation of the cognitively impaired (Sinason, 1992).

Two recent pieces of research are worth mentioning here, as they relate specifically to the provision of hospice care. Hogg *et al*'s research (2001) into how people with learning disabilities access cancer services showed significant inequalities across the range of services, from cancer screening through to end-of-life care. Sadly, they showed that not only were people with learning disabilities less likely to access palliative care at all, but also that they were further discriminated against in that they routinely failed to access the full range of services available within the resource to which they were referred. Thus, although a person with a learning disability may rarely be referred to a hospice, even when they did so they were unlikely to be offered day hospice placements or complementary therapy sessions.

Research funded by the UK Foundation for People with Learning Disabilities and carried out by Professor Brown of the Salomons Centre (University of Canterbury, UK) highlighted the differences in palliative-care provision for people with learning disabilities when they had a diagnosis of dementia, as opposed to a cancer diagnosis. There were striking differences in the levels of specialist provision available and in the coordination of services. This would lead one to conclude that a person with a learning disability and dementia would not only be doubly disadvantaged at the end of their life, but potentially triply disadvantaged. The implications for the service user are obvious, but it is clear from this research also that care staff pay a high price for trying to ensure a 'good death' for their service user in the face of the scarcest of resources (Brown *et al*, 2003).

The role of the hospice

What then is the role of the hospice in caring for people with learning disabilities who experience life-threatening illness? A recent definition of palliative care asserts that:

Palliative care is an approach that improves the quality of the life of patients and their families facing the problems associated with life-threatening illness, through the prevention and relief of suffering by means of early identification and impeccable assessment and treatment of pain and other problems physical, psychosocial and spiritual.

(WHO, 2003).

In keeping with this, it would seem that there is a role for the hospice as advocate, assessor and controller of symptoms (including the physical, emotional and spiritual), as well as a carer for the family, a supporter and educator of staff and, ultimately, as a learner. This is perhaps best illustrated by a case study.

Case Study 11.1: Sophie's story

Sophie was in her early forties when she was referred to a hospice community nursing service of an independent hospice. Some months before, she had been diagnosed with bowel cancer and secondary spread to her liver. Because no further treatment had been recommended, her case was considered to be incurable, although death was not imminent.

At the time of diagnosis, Sophie was living in a medium-secure unit for people with a dual diagnosis of learning disability and mental-health problems. She had previously spent some time in the prison system and her behaviour was considered to be both challenging and at times violent. She was several hundred miles from her family primarily because a specialist resource, such as the one she was living in, was not available in her home area.

The first visit to Sophie was a joint visit by a Macmillan nurse and a palliative care social worker. Although the purpose of the visit was to meet Sophie, very little time was spent with her, but rather more time was spent with the multidisciplinary team (including the psychologist and learning-disability and mental-health nurses) who gave the history of Sophie's diagnosis.

Sophie, it became clear, had been unwell for a number of months. She had seen her GP to complain of stomach pain on several occasions, and had even been seen by her local hospital. Nothing had been found that might explain her level of discomfort, and there had been concern about a potentially 'attention-seeking' element to her 'illness'. Over the course of one weekend, Sophie had become very unwell and continually screamed out in pain. She was eventually admitted to hospital where physicians discovered that she was in bowel obstruction and would require immediate surgery. Physicians also discovered that, at some point in the past few months, her bowel had both ruptured and healed over. The staff were shocked at the seriousness of the illness and the fact that her previous complaints of pain had been very much underplayed, given the trauma she had been through. They felt very guilty that they had underestimated the gravity of her situation.

An interview with the surgeon revealed that in addition to the bowel cancer, he had also identified two areas of cancer spread in her liver. He had not suggested any further curative treatment and in response to staff questioning had confirmed that Sophie would die from this illness. Staff had decided to tell Sophie the truth, but had cautioned her against telling fellow residents for fear that they may tease or bully her about this.

At the time of referral, staff wanted help to assess and control Sophie's pain, help with telling the other residents, with supporting Sophie, and with dealing with the news themselves. They were very keen to keep Sophie with them until the end of her life, but were aware that this may prove impossible.

When the nurse and social worker finally met with Sophie, she expressed a desire to have someone help her with the pain and also to have someone to talk to about what was happening to her. She was clearly very frightened and feared that her death would be both painful and imminent.

Hospice as advocate

At the first visit, it became obvious to the nurse and social worker that there were some surprising elements to Sophie's story which related to treatment decisions. Given her relatively young age, it was unusual to hear that the surgeon had made a decision not to refer Sophie onto an oncologist for assessment of the merits of curative treatment. Certainly it would be usual for such a patient to be offered surgical removal of the liver metastases (secondary cancers) with the aim of prolonging her life.

On presentation later at the community palliative care meeting, this scenario was explored and the palliative care doctor agreed to present Sophie's case at a joint surgery and oncology meeting, which he duly did. In the event, it did not change the decision and Sophie was not offered any chemotherapy on the basis that it was unlikely to change her prognosis greatly and may indeed have reduced further her quality of life in the last months. However, this discussion was an important one and although it may not have achieved a different outcome for Sophie, it is likely that it will have influenced the future care of other patients with learning disabilities in that hospital.

The role of advocacy is not a new one for hospices that have developed over many years in an almost counter-cultural context. Historically, the focus of advocacy has been around the withdrawal of 'futile' treatments. Indeed, it was Cicely Saunders's observation of numerous patients undergoing harsh treatments long past any efficacy (because doctors with nothing else to offer felt they were abandoning their patients) that caused her to set up St Christopher's. The hospice became a place where patients could have some respite from treatment and gave carers an opportunity to undertake the emotional work associated with dying.

In relation to people with learning disabilities, the hospice has a role as advocate in ensuring that such patients are given the same options as those who do not have a cognitive disability. This is likely to include access to services, for it is not uncommon to hear of community services refusing to visit because the person lives in a group home. In part, this is due to a lack of understanding that learning-disability nursing is primarily a social model of nursing as opposed to the traditional model. Confronted with limited resources, a district nurse may respond by saying that if there are 'nursing' staff in the home, the patients' needs will be met without her involvement.

However, it is clear that the hospice cannot advocate for the patient unless it has first put its own house in order. Fortunately, this area of practice in hospice care is developing and is backed by a commitment and interest from those organisations responsible for the development of policy and standards within the hospice movement (eg. Help the Hospices and the National Council for Hospice and Palliative Care), to say nothing of individual professional associations that seem now to be taking this issue on (eg. The Royal College of Nursing [RCN]).

Hospice as multidisciplinary assessor

Integral to the concept of palliative care is the idea that both assessment and intervention are the activities of a multidisciplinary team. At the first visit with Sophie, several issues arose, including:

- Placement issues. Impediments to staying in the present accommodation included registration status, ie. not being registered for the nursing care that Sophie was likely to need progressively.
- The impact of Sophie's illness on other residents. This was a particular consideration in the medium secure unit where other residents' mental health was likely to be affected by knowledge of Sophie's illness, and where any mental instability may result in challenging behaviour. If this were directed at Sophie, it could place her in a vulnerable position, especially given her physical condition.
- The impact on staff and their ability to manage the competing demands of Sophie's condition and that of the other residents.

It became clear that Sophie was likely to need help with:

- Deciding where she wanted to spend her last days of life.
- Reviewing her life in a positive way that acknowledged her achievements, many of which had taken place in the past few months.
- Thinking about issues related to her family relationships. Sophie expressed a need to think about what she wanted to leave her family members when she died. She had said that she wanted to make a will, which, given her learning disability and her mental health section, was unlikely to be straightforward.
- Speaking about her illness with other residents of her choice.
- Symptom control and being able to discuss her fears with people who could handle the intensity of emotion this was likely to generate.

For the staff, there were several needs also:

- To understand the likely progression of Sophie's illness, including being able to distinguish significant issues whilst dispelling fantasies.
- To be able to understand emotional responses to loss generally and in relation to Sophie particularly.
- To devise strategies to deal with their own emotions.
- To devise strategies to deal with Sophie's questions consistently whilst taking account of staff members' differing abilities to deal with death and dying.
- To become aware of the various agencies and professionals who were likely to become involved.
- To devise ways of dealing with other residents' distress and questions in response to Sophie's progressing illness.

Some of the very practical issues concerned:

- Placement — types, locations and funding of alternative placements should it prove impossible for Sophie to stay in the unit.
- Financial issues — including benefits available to Sophie because of her diagnosed terminal illness and accessing of grants for Sophie to enable her mother to visit.
- Differing models of care — deciding who needs to be involved in Sophie's care at each stage, given her physical and mental health needs and learning disability.
- Issues likely to arise as a result of the mental-health section.

An initial programme of action included:

- To check out hospice provision in the area where her family lived and whether they would be able to cope with both the learning disability and mental-health needs.
- To search for literature for staff around palliative care, bereavement and palliative-care needs.

- Checking out the situation with regard to registration and the legality of Sophie being able to remain in her present home throughout the progression of her disease.
- Clarification of staff training and support needs.
- Clarifying whether the emotional support of Sophie and other residents could be provided by the unit staff, or whether it would need to be provided by the hospice team.
- Setting up an initial appointment with a palliative-care physician to undertake a thorough assessment of Sophie's physical care and symptom-control needs.

Hospice as symptom control

The primary reason that most people are referred to the hospice is for the assessment and treatment of 'intractable symptoms'. It would be true to say that the community focus tends to be on the physical symptoms such as pain and nausea. However, within the hospice, there is a more holistic assessment of the elements of what Cicely Saunders has called 'total pain' (Saunders, 1964).

Saunders developed the concept of total pain to signify that for many confronting terminal illness, the most difficult issues are not physical but may be psychological, social, emotional or spiritual. In Sophie's situation, this was certainly true, although all these elements have a part to play, physical pain (or its absence) is often the primary factor in determining quality of life. Therefore, one of the first things that was undertaken was the assessment of physical pain and other symptoms. This was not straightforward for Sophie, who complained of pain throughout her body. Asked if she had pain in her big toe (as an attempt to ease the situation with some light humour), she confirmed that she did indeed have pain in her big toe, although the reason why remained unclear.

For Sophie, as for many others, there was a close association between the words 'cancer', 'pain' and 'death', which was fuelled by past experience of having seen a relative die in extreme pain from a gastric cancer. Therefore, it seemed that when Sophie felt pain she feared death, and as she feared death, so her physical sensation of pain increased. This had obviously heightened subsequent to the diagnosis of cancer in that she had previously undergone the rupture and healing of her bowel without expressing the level of pain that she did now, post-diagnosis. However, there were some simple things such as analgesics and complementary therapies that, at this stage, improved Sophie's discomfort; these, in conjunction with coming to trust and understand her new environment, enabled her to spend most of her illness in a relatively pain-free condition. Sophie's case demonstrates well the psychological aspects of pain — ie. the meaning one attributes to pain can intensify or alleviate it. This effect might be especially complex for someone with a learning disability, in that the meaning attributed to the pain is not always readily accessible either to the sufferer nor to those who seek to help them.

Many people with a learning disability do not perceive a causal relationship between illness and death; others have an exaggerated sense of it, so they are fearful of a cold because they think it might kill them (McEvoy, 1989). Like many of us, they are also influenced by what is said by those whom they trust. Sophie had asked a carer, 'What is dying like?' The carer, trying to be gentle with her, had replied, 'I don't know. I suppose it's a bit like sleeping'. Understandably, Sophie then spent many weeks afraid of going to sleep.

We too tried to explain the progression of illness to Sophie in a simple, non-dramatic way, explaining to her that she would progressively lose weight, get more sleepy and weak. This, however, proved so frightening to Sophie (because she was already tired, weaker and had lost some weight) that our physician broke all the rules of his training and assured Sophie that she was not dying just now, but that when she was he would tell her. Although we were worried about taking this approach, our justification was that it seemed to ease Sophie's fears and enable her to change focus.

In time, Sophie's understanding of her pain developed. On one occasion, having been admitted from the nursing home where she had screamed in pain continually for twenty-four hours, Sophie was given analgesia and sedation. The cause of her pain was found to be bone metastases, which required radiotherapy. As Sophie's pain was controlled and her sedation reduced, I was able to talk to her about her pain and what had happened. I asked her, 'When you were screaming, was it because you were in pain or because you were frightened?' to which she answered, 'Bit of both really'. It became clear that Sophie had experienced a new type of pain, and this had sent her back into a cycle whereby she came to believe that she was now dying and this fear had increased her pain (both physically and mentally) such that it had spiralled out of control.

Sophie's ability to understand her illness also developed, which is often the case in other people with learning disabilities. It is almost as if there is a time-lag in understanding, which is resolved by concrete experience of seeing others who are ill around you. For Sophie, this was also achieved by watching a film in which a young girl had died of cancer after a decision had been taken by doctors not to remove a tumour from her stomach. Sophie now remembered that there were bits of her cancer that had not been cut out at the time of her surgery, and she began to ask whether she could have these removed now.

It is very difficult to disentangle the emotional dimension of one's pain from the physical dimension. In the words of Parkes (1979), 'pain is a psycho-biological phenomenon', although palliative-care professionals recognise that not all emotional pain can be resolved. Earnshaw-Smith (1982) explored the concept of emotional pain more than twenty years ago, but her findings have as much relevance to our present work as they did then. In summary, she postulated that emotional pain is:

- experienced in the present is closely interwoven with the pain of the past
- is inextricably linked with physical pain
- can arise out of misconceptions
- is subjective
- though unacceptable is an appropriate response to the situation
- is often caused by fear, the unknown and the unpredictable
- is often caused by remorse and guilt and is intensified by separation and loss (Earnshaw-Smith, 1982).

For Sophie, her previous ways of dealing with such pain were to injure others and most often herself; it is a vindication of the palliative care approach that, although she did at times fantasise about hurting or killing herself, she attempted neither. In time, Sophie became able to hold within herself the distress she was experiencing until she was able to explore it with one of the small group of people identified to help her with this.

Hospice as spiritual care

One of the most neglected areas of care of people with learning disabilities is spiritual care. One of the great strengths of the hospice movement has been to see spiritual care as a core service — part of addressing that total pain spectrum. Research by Swinton (2001) has shown that spiritual concerns are as important to people with learning disabilities as those without, although they may be expressed differently.

Family and spiritual-care concerns were inextricably linked for Sophie. Her life had been a complicated one: she had spent time within the penal system and was not allowed to make contact with some members of her family; she was under mental-health section and at times was aggressive and violent. Having been told that she would die from her cancer, Sophie expressed fear over what came after death for someone such as she. One of the very important relationships she made then was with the chaplain.

On a visit from the social worker, Sophie recounted a conversation that had taken place on the previous evening. Sophie had been in pain and was crying and fearful. A nurse had come to her room and had tried to deal with her pain and in the course of the conversation had told Sophie that she prayed for her daily. Sophie's response had been quite alarmed and she said, 'You mustn't do that!'

For Sophie, there was a sense of shame expressed as the idea that she was somehow beyond the pale of people's prayers, and even that someone praying for her may somehow get them into trouble, though from whom was unclear. This was probably related to Sophie's sense of what she had done wrong in her life, which had resulted in her being in prison or in hospital. However, as with other learning-disabled people, her sense of shame may well have originated in her disability. Some feel ashamed of having made life so tough (as they see it) for their parents simply by virtue of their existence. One man said, 'Mum would have been all right; she would have had a good life it hadn't been for me'.

Sophie was also concerned that she would not be welcomed in 'heaven' when she died because, amongst other things, she had not been baptised. The chaplain explained to Sophie that people were not barred from heaven solely on the basis of having been baptised or not. However, it was clear to him that she understood the concept and wanted baptism as a sign of her forgiveness by God. Thus, she requested that she be baptised in the hospice chapel — to which the chaplain agreed. She drew up an invitation list to her baptism, and was strict in her requirements that women must not wear trousers but must wear hats! Photographs had to be taken of all involved, and a reception afterwards was hosted by the unit in which she lived.

One could be forgiven for believing that Sophie just wanted a party. But although it was clear that the party was very important to her, so too was the baptism itself. During the ritual, Sophie laughed and cried at appropriate moments. Gathered around her were many of her family members, one of whom was greatly relieved that Sophie had undergone baptism; to her, it was a sign that Sophie had understood the many religious services to which she had been taken during her life. It seemed that something very important had taken place for Sophie in her relationship with God, and also in terms of trying to 'put right' an earlier stage of her life, which she had been powerless to do until then.

Another issue in the process of being explored in the literature is the sense among learning-disabled people that they won't be remembered when they die. Of course, there is good reason for them to feel this way; as both Todd (2002) and Blackman (2003) point out, there are few remembering rituals for people with learning disabilities, and most members of the public expect family members to view the death as a 'blessed release' rather than a full-blown bereavement. However, this is an issue of importance in palliative care. How does one care for someone who must, at some level, view their dying as the fulfilment of the wish that society has expressed towards them since their birth? How can they mourn their own passing when they remain unsure about whether the world will?

Sophie had this anxiety too, but it was addressed through intuitive, specialised caring. On one occasion, Sophie told the social worker that the unit she lived in had planted a tree in the garden by which to remember her. For Sophie, this was a very reassuring symbol that people would continue to remember her after she had died. It was also important because she knew then that the other residents who did not know that she was going to die would remember her too.

Sophie decided that she wanted to plan her funeral. She had not attended any funerals in her life and so requested that she visit the crematorium. She also took the opportunity to speak with the organist and to have him play her funeral hymns in her hearing. She told him that he had better 'play them right' on the day, as she would looking down on him and would come back to haunt him if he did not. The funeral that had just left when she arrived had many floral tributes and it was Sophie's assessment that this meant that the person had been loved greatly. Thereafter, she did not fail to tell people that she wanted flowers at her funeral!

Hospice as carer for the family

Largest of all the differences between care in other settings and in the hospice is the degree of support offered to family (or significant others of the patient). The greater support offered in the hospice is at the heart of palliative care, and indeed features in earlier definitions of palliative care as 'the family forms the unit of care', which is to say that the whole family is the client, not just the patient (National Council for Hospice and Specialist Palliative Care, 1995).

It is clear that one of the most effective ways to care for the patient is to offer care to the whole family. Outside the confines of the hospice, it may seem strange to be telling someone how you will work with their loved ones after their death. However, this is often very reassuring and can enable the patient to let go of their life more peacefully if they are sure that their loved ones or dependants will continue to be cared for after their death.

Research by Kissane and Bloch (2002) has identified a positive correlation between the pre-morbid functioning of the family unit and bereavement outcome. It has been found that families whose level of function and communication was poor before the death are more likely to experience complicated bereavement reactions. This highlights the need for a proactive approach. Kissane and Bloch's work promotes a useful systemic approach that fits well with the adage that 'cancer affects many more people than it infects'.

The palliative-care perspective asserts that it is the patient who defines who constitutes 'family' and therefore the provision of support is extended to all those who are so identified by the patient and who wish to avail themselves of the service. In the case of the person with a learning disability, this may just as likely be a fellow resident as a sibling.

In Sophie's case, the support of the family was at a distance. Sophie's life had been complicated, it seemed, right from birth and her family was a very fractured one. Some siblings had retained a close and caring relationship with her; others had a less positive relationship with her; and others had no relationship with her at all. She had retained a strong bond with her mother, but was aware that her mother was also the mother of those siblings who were less positive towards her. Initially, Sophie looked to her mother for a great deal of emotional support. Later, with Sophie concerned about the impact her dying was having on her mother, their relationship was almost reversed.

Sadly, though Sophie had a number of months in which to achieve a resolution of some of her relationships, the situation was not completely in her control. Therefore, as there were family members to whom she was not able to express her love physically, work was done to help her create 'memory boxes' that could be given after her death. Hopefully, this had a positive effect on the bereavement of those receiving them. But even if it did not, it was important for Sophie to enact that resolution within herself and to have the opportunity to explore the issues while fantasising both about receiving the forgiveness of her loved ones, and what life might have been like had things been different. This, I believe, was an important part of Sophie's ability to let go of her life when the time came to do so.

Hospice as staff supporter

The holistic care of people with learning disabilities renders staff confronting terminal illness in one of their clients in need of a great deal of support. It is one thing to apply to work in a hospice, where death is an almost daily occurrence; but many people are attracted to the care of people with learning disabilities precisely because they want to work with the living. However, given that there are now few long-stay learning-disability hospitals (and soon will be none), this is going to be an increasing problem in working with an ageing learning-disability population.

Presently, the cultures of most learning-disability establishments are 'death-denying' — ie. they behave as if dying and bereavement either do not happen or are to be avoided at all costs. This is for a number of reasons, in part to do with the age profile of most learning-disability carers, and the fact that they may not have had much experience of death and dying themselves. Todd has recently undertaken a thorough analysis of these reasons (Todd, 2002).

In Sophie's situation the staff were very committed to caring for her and initially intended that she should remain in the unit until her death. However, huge levels of staff anxiety and sadness accompanied this. The anxiety was about the impact Sophie's death would have on other residents and whether they would be able to cope with that as well as their own feelings.

Their feelings were intense and related in part to a series of personal bereavements of staff members, including the death of both a member of staff and another service-user. They were also related to the fact that, by dint of their hard work and Sophie's cooperation, they had achieved great things for Sophie such that it was likely that she would have been discharged from the unit back into the community in less than a year. It was difficult for staff to view Sophie's death as anything other than unfair. It was impossible for them to see her death at this stage as something that she could achieve, in keeping with her other achievements, rather than in contrast to them.

There were several pragmatic issues related to the registration status of the unit (ie. residential and not nursing), as well as management issues in terms of how to deal with Sophie's mental health should it deteriorate. For instance, one of the questions that was raised was whether control and restraint measures could be used on Sophie should her mental health deteriorate. It is clear that for someone who could at any time develop cancer bone secondaries, this would be inadvisable — but, for the unit, so was the prospect of failing to respond consistently to challenging behaviour expressed by any of their residents.

The Macmillan nurse, palliative-care social worker and palliative-care doctor organised three training sessions. The organisation provided cover so that almost all staff could attend the sessions, out of which guidelines for Sophie's care were to be developed. The sessions included information on cancer and its likely progression; the control of pain and other symptoms; the emotional aspects of being terminally ill and some information about bereavement. Sessions were managed openly to allow for the expression of staff members' own perspectives on Sophie's illness and the impact on them both as individuals and as a staff group. In addition, where members of staff found it particularly hard, counselling and supervision were offered.

In the event, the unit was not able to retain the care of Sophie. Once her mental-health section was lifted, it became increasingly hard to justify her continued placement in the unit — especially given that there were several hazards that Sophie would encounter on a daily basis from other residents, whose mental health rendered them incapable of understanding why Sophie might have (as they saw it) preferential treatment.

Sophie spent her last days between a nursing home and the hospice. Once moved to the nursing home, a similar programme of training and support for nursing-home staff was set up. For these staff, who were mainly young and inexperienced, the issues were their distress at someone so young dying when most of their elderly residents were likely to live for some time. There were also issues for some of the staff in being able to understand the learning disability and the mental-health problems. Furthermore, as Sophie began to trust them and talk about her life, some found the details of her life very distressing. Eventually, the hospice staff worked with Sophie to enable her to limit her frankest discussion to those people who were able to cope with what they were likely to hear.

After Sophie's death, a debriefing session was held with the nursing home staff to facilitate the expression of their own feelings.

Hospice as educator

Education is linked to the issue of staff support. From the earliest days of the hospice movement, education has been an integral part of influencing care. Most hospice staff, therefore, will have a commitment to educate and most hospices will have a robust education programme.

As palliative care has moved away from the care of those exclusively with a diagnosis of cancer, so has its teaching. It is now commonplace to find education about conditions such as Parkinson's disease, motor neurone disease, HIV/AIDS. In addition, a number of the staple topics have transferable value, irrespective of the diagnosis, eg. communication, breaking bad news and bereavement courses.

Some hospices have begun to take the needs of the learning-disabled population seriously and provide education to support this. It is also likely that even if a hospice is not presently providing such courses, there will nevertheless be hospice staff who would be capable of delivering these, perhaps in partnership with their local learning-disability colleagues. Where partnerships do not exist and the local hospice is unable to provide relevant courses, an organisation such as The National Network for the Palliative Care of People with Learning Disabilities should be able to provide information about people who are providing training either locally or through the Network national study days.

Hospice as learner

At the end of the year, Sophie attended the hospice carol service. Her pain was well-controlled and she was excited at the prospect of finally getting her electric wheelchair and being able, as a result, to go on holiday. The following week she was visited as usual by the trainee counsellor, by which time the wheelchair had arrived and she was learning to use it whilst helping the nurses to decorate the Christmas tree.

A few days later, Sophie was found in her room quietly crying. When the staff asked what was wrong, she told them that she wasn't going to be around for much longer. A few days later still, when her family visited her, she also told them she was going to die soon. Naturally concerned, they asked whether her condition had changed, which in fact it had not, and although Sophie was deteriorating, it was happening fairly slowly. However, shortly after this visit, Sophie did indeed deteriorate more rapidly. It had been her expressed wish throughout that she wanted to die in the hospice. She was admitted on a Saturday afternoon and died there peacefully within twelve hours.

Sophie's funeral was conducted as requested by the Chaplain, strictly according to her wishes. There were many family members there, plus staff from all the settings in which she had spent her final months. Almost without exception, those who attended brought flowers. The hymn, which Sophie had chosen, was 'Amazing Grace'.

Final thoughts

What did we learn In response to this question, we could simultaneously answer 'nothing new' and 'everything afresh'. Sophie reminded us of the importance of multidisciplinary working; of recognising the different elements of total pain; and of responding to each appropriately. She taught us anew the importance of spiritual care for all those confronting their death, including people with learning disabilities. For Sophie, her spiritual needs had the 'loudest' voice and the resolution of her spiritual distress was evident in the words of her funeral hymn — 'Amazing grace how sweet the sound that saved a wretch like me…' — chosen by her as someone whose literal sense was more strongly developed than her abstract sense. She reminded us powerfully that palliative care done well enables not only life review, but a resolution of life's events that enables us to die peacefully.

Above all, Sophie reminded us that, however skilled we are, the patient remains the expert on both their life and on their dying. In *The Platform Ticket* (1999), Derek Doyle describes how we, as professionals, might buy the platform ticket that enables us to travel some of the way alongside dying people, helping them with pieces of luggage they must either carry or leave behind; but, crucially, Doyle also reminds us that, in the end, they must take that final part of the journey alone. We had believed that, out of kindness, we would tell Sophie when that final stage in the journey had come and would try to make it easier for her. But, as our patients often do irrespective of cognitive ability, Sophie instead told us, and made the parting all the harder. Somehow, however, she also left us with the sense that she had achieved in her dying what she had sought for all her life — the concrete evidence that her life had mattered.

References

Blackman N, Todd S (2003) *Caring for People with Learning Disabilities who are Dying.* Worth Publishing, London

Blackman N (2003) *Learning Disability and Bereavement.* Worth Publishing, London

Blackman N (ed) (2000) *Living with Loss: Helping People with Learning Disabilities Cope with Bereavement and Loss.* Pavilion Publishing, Brighton

Brown H, Burns S, Flynn M (2005) *Dying Matters.* London Salomons Centre Kent & Foundation for People with Learning Disabilities

DoH (2003) *Supportive and Palliative Care.* Information sheet on palliative care and hospices. Section 4. DoH, London

DoH (2001) *Valuing People: a New Strategy for Learning Disability for the 21st Century.* Government White Paper. DoH, London

DoH (1998) *Signposts for Success in Commissioning and Providing Health Services for People with Learning Disabilities.* Wetherby. DoH, London

DoH (1995) *The Health of the Nation: a Strategy for People with Learning Disability.* HMSO, London

Doyle D (1999) *The Platform Ticket: Memories and Musings of a Hospice Doctor.* Pentland Press, Durham

Earnshaw-Smith E (1982) Emotional pain in dying patients and their families. *Nurs Times* **78**(44): 1865–7

Hogg J, Northfield J, Turnbull J (2001) *Cancer and People with Learning Disabilities: the Evidence from Published Studies and Experiences from Cancer Services.* BILD, Kidderminster

Hospice Information Service (HIS) (2003) *Hospice and Palliative Care Facts and Figures* (2003). HIS, London

Kissane DW, Bloch S (2002) *Family Focused Grief Therapy.* Open University Press, London

McEnhill L (2004) In: Oliviere D, Monroe B (eds) *Death, Dying and Social Difference.* Oxford

University Press, Oxford

McEnhill L (2005) Specialist palliative care social work with people who have learning disabilities. In: Parker J (ed) *Aspects of Social Work and Palliative Care*. Quay Books, London

McEvoy J (1989) Investigating the concept of death in adults who are mentally handicapped. *Br J Mental Subnormal* **35**(2): 69

National Council for Hospice and Specialist Palliative Care (1995) *Specialist Palliative Care: a Statement of Definitions*. Occasional Paper No. 7, London

Parkes CM (1979) Terminal care: evaluation of inpatient service at St Christopher's Hospice Part 1: views of surviving spouse on effects of the service on the patient. *Postgrad Med J* **55**: 517–22

Saunders C (1964) Care of patients suffering from terminal illness at St Joseph's Hospice, Hackney, London. *Nurs Mirror* **14 Feb**: vii–x

Shorter Oxford English Dictionary (1988) Guild Publishing, London

Sinason V (1992) *Mental Handicap and the Human Condition: New Approaches from the Tavistock*. Free Association Books, London

Swinton J (2001) *A Space to Listen: Meeting the Spiritual Needs of People with Learning Disabilities*. The Mental Health Foundation, London

The National Network for the Palliative Care of People with Learning Disabilities. St Nicholas Hospice, Macmillan Way, Hardwick Lane, Bury St Edmunds, Suffolk IP33 2QY, UK (www.helpthehospices.org.uk)

Todd S (2002) Death does not become us: the absence of death and dying in intellectual disability research. *J Gerontol Soc Work* **38**: 225–39

World Health Organisation (WHO) (2003) (www.who.int/cancer/palliative/definition/en/)

CHAPTER 11

Research, palliative care and learning disability

Edward Lindop

The intention of this chapter is to explore some of the main principles of the three major research paradigms — quantitative, qualitative and triangulation — that govern research thinking today. An attempt will also be made to review these in the light of sensitive research, especially research associated with palliative care. Research methods used within each of the paradigms will be considered in the context of learning disabilities. An implicit theme within the chapter is the deficiency in service provision for people with learning disabilities and, in particular, those who are in need of palliative care.

Belief systems

Human belief systems are the basis of our understanding of the universe and evolution. This is illustrated in history by the belief that the world was flat and that to continue to travel beyond the horizon would mean eventually falling off the end of the world. It took an enormous leap of faith to look beyond this and to accommodate the view that the world was round, but the leap of faith was made with the help of science and innovation.

Religion provides another example of the profound effects of belief in our everyday life. People over the ages have fought wars and tolerated human suffering beyond appreciation in the name of their particular religious belief. Different people have different beliefs. These may be related to a belief in oneself, another person, or a social system. A particular belief system can profoundly direct someone's life, as can be seen in the case of various religions, where people can murder with impunity or sacrifice their life without hesitation in the name of their religious belief.

Research paradigms

A belief system can extend beyond a belief in religion and can be related to almost anything. For instance, a person may have a superstitious belief that opening an umbrella in the house is bad luck, or that if a friend gives you a knife as a present, you should cross their palm with money so that the knife will not sever the friendship.

Belief systems in research are referred to as paradigms. A research paradigm can govern the way in which a researcher operates. If a researcher totally believes in a particular paradigm, he or she may be unable to accept that there are alternative models of research, just as the person who believed that the world was flat could not accept that it was round. There are three dominant research paradigms:

■ The scientific paradigm, commonly referred to as the 'quantitative paradigm' and also known as 'positivism' (which is the term that will be used in this chapter hereafter).
■ The alternative paradigm, often referred to as the 'qualitative paradigm'.
■ Triangulation, a new belief system or paradigm that has emerged more recently.

The positivist paradigm

The oldest research paradigm is the positivist paradigm, which has its routes in the science tradition. The positivist believes that universal laws, which are just as profound as the law of gravitation or other physical laws, govern the world. However, the positivist believes that this law can be applied to social systems and human behaviour. This law is the law of probability which, according to the positivist, relates to the probability of any event occurring or not occurring. In short, at one end of the chance continuum is certainty — for example, death — while at the other is the chance of an event being remote — for example, winning the lottery. The positivist argues that all events in life can be measured in relation to their chance of occurring or not occurring, and this concept can be applied to the potential for one event being responsible for causing or influencing a second event — for example, constant frustration causing anger.

The measurement tool used to determine the probability of an event occurring or not occurring is statistics. However, to be able to determine whether or not one thing has been the cause of another, all other happenings around the event have to be controlled. For example, if you wish to claim that effective communication before surgery improves recovery following surgery, you have to show that it is effective communication and not other factors that have been responsible for the improvement. To apply statistical measurement to events or behaviour, the behaviour in question has to be reduced to its lowest form. This always involves the use of numbers, so all events or behaviours being researched are represented numerically, with a particular cut-off point signifying that one event, such as effective communication before surgery, did (or did not) cause more rapid improvement following surgery. The positivist believes that applying strict laws of science will enable generalisation that a statistically significant finding in one setting will also be found in a similar setting. For instance, if effective communication before surgery has been shown to improve recovery following surgery in one hospital, then it should in a second hospital, providing that nothing has 'contaminated the experiment'.

The qualitative paradigm

The qualitative paradigm rejects the assumptions embodied in positivism, claiming that concepts such as experimental control and statistical analysis are more appropriate for laboratory experiments, but are unrelated to the real world of human behaviour and interaction. Unlike the positivist paradigm, this paradigm implies that the only way to gain answers to research questions related to human behaviour is to examine them in context — that is, in their natural environment. Therefore, importance is placed on the uniqueness of the individual and understanding their world, rather than reducing understanding to an examination of chance through statistical analysis. The qualitative paradigm, then, is inductive rather than deductive. It seeks to understand the human experience in the context of social interaction — for example, understanding how communities function by understanding the individual's experience within it. This runs contrary to positivism, which is deductive in that it attempts to express statistically human interaction within a community.

Triangulation

The third paradigm is triangulation. A traditional research description of triangulation would be mixed methods — that is, using both quantitative and qualitative methods in a single study. However, the origins of triangulation can be found in cartography, meaning three points on a map, or in research terms, looking at things from three different perspectives. However, in more recent times, triangulation has come to mean approaching research from different perspectives. For example, using both quantitative and qualitative methods (method triangulation); using different researchers (researcher triangulation); or analysing data using a number of different data-analysis techniques. Arguments about the strengths and weaknesses of triangulation persist. On the one hand, it is said to confuse the issue in that it does not present a clear epistemology (knowledge-base); on the other, the claim is that it increases validity because it approaches the research from a number of different perspectives.

Sensitive research

The appropriate paradigm to use in different healthcare research is an extremely important consideration. Indeed, McCarthy (1998: 140) argues that 'choosing the appropriate method for the task is itself an ethical issue'. Healthcare research can also be predominantly classified as sensitive research since the people being researched are often vulnerable. This is another important issue to consider in terms of which method to use. Sensitive topics also raise difficult methodological problems, which is illustrated by Townsend *et al* (1990) when interviewing terminally ill people in relation to their preferred place of death and final care.

Before examining the issue of which research methods based on which research paradigms might be appropriate for sensitive research tasks, it is useful to consider definitions of sensitive research. Lee (1995: 2) defines sensitive research in a simple way, stating that 'a simple definition of sensitive research would therefore be research which potentially poses a substantial threat to those who are or have been involved in it'. A more all-embracing definition, however, is offered by Owen (2001: 656): 'Research is to be considered sensitive when the people being studied are powerless or disadvantaged, where there is an opportunity for people to feel exploited or degraded, or where the subject matter is related to personal experience'.

Descriptions of people being disadvantaged, vulnerable, powerless or exploited raise the question — should people in those situations be involved in research? McCarthy (1998: 140) provides a direct answer, arguing that 'certain areas of human life are too sensitive to be researched and therefore ought not to be'. If these definitions were to be adopted by the research community, it would be virtually impossible to pursue research in the healthcare setting because it could be argued that everyone who is ill is vulnerable in one way or another.

However, these definitions look toward the negative aspects of investigation and, as McCarthy (1998) notes, negative views of harmful effects of research neglect the positive aspects. Indeed, there are beneficial experiences for research participants, even where sensitive research is concerned. For example, Townsend *et al* (1990) show that research of sensitive topics can be cathartic for research participants and their families. They also go on to show that studies involving sensitive research challenge taken-for-granted ways of seeing the world and are important precisely because the research illuminates the darker corners of society. White and Barnitt (200) concede that there may be unacceptable risks in being a subject in a socially sensitive research project, but avoiding research among people with learning disability would mean that their voices would not be heard. Atkinson (1988) also shows that people with learning disabilites were able to contribute to research projects that focused on their lifestyle.

Research methods and palliative care

Research into palliative care is one of the best examples of sensitive research that meets all the criteria in the definition by Owen (2001). Yet a considerable number of projects have been undertaken in palliative care using all the main paradigms previously described. Palliative care is concerned with quality of life rather than cure, and pertains to physical, social, psychological and spiritual well-being. Positivist methods seem to be inappropriate in palliative care, with many people arguing that a method purporting a scientific approach is incompatible with a situation requiring compassionate care. A reduction of feelings and emotions to a statistical analysis does seem inappropriate when the primary objective is to provide holistic care, rather than a blunt intrusion into the remaining life of people with terminal illness.

Yet, leaving the ethical debate aside, successful quantitative studies have been undertaken. For example, Addington-Hall *et al* (1992) examined the effects on terminally ill cancer patients and their families of coordinating the services available within the NHS and from local authorities plus the voluntary sector. For this they allocated 554 patients with a survival expectancy of less than one year to a control or experimental group. The coordination group of patients received the assistance of two nurse coordinators, whose role was to ensure that patients in their group received appropriate and well-coordinated services, tailored to their individual needs and circumstances.

However, while the research project could be considered successful from a design perspective, is it either ethical or morally appropriate to use control and experimental groups where one group of terminally ill people receive potentially better care than another?

Lee (1995: 119) puts forward a view that 'field research based on qualitative methods such as participant observation or depth interviewing has often seemed like the method of choice in studying sensitive research'. However, interviewing patients during their last days of life can be intrusive. Many patients are too ill or too fatigued to participate by the time they are receiving palliative care. Indeed, in the study by Addington-Hall *et al* (1992), 35% of a group of patients with cancer and a life expectancy of less than one year died before they could be interviewed. This view is supported by Cannon (1989: 64) who undertook research associated with the study of women's experiences of treatment for breast cancer:

It was obvious, for example, that survey methods and questionnaires would not yield the information I required. Similarly, there was no way of conducting the research covertly, nor had I any desire to do so. I felt that, clearly, the success of the research depended upon my being able to form relationships with women which would involve, at the very least, gaining their confidence and trust which would, in turn, necessitate some emotional input on my part in the relationship.

An important point to consider in this statement is the reference to an 'input' on the part of the researcher. The positivist would see this as being a way of contaminating the research findings because forming relationships with participants and gaining their confidence would amount to a lack of experimental control (making the findings of the research unreliable and invalid). The point made by Cannon is supported by McCarthy (1998: 141) who interviewed seventeen women with learning disabilities on the subject of their sexual experiences (the women all had mild-to-moderate learning disability). McCarthy draws attention to the researcher's personal vulnerability as well as the research participant's:

When the women did ask me questions, they were occasionally about whether I engaged in specific sexual activities. This was a sobering reminder that even when it is your job to talk and to write about sex all day, as mine had been for several years now, it is quite a different matter to talk about your own sex life.

These examples highlight the fact that when undertaking sensitive research, both the participant and the researcher are vulnerable and, according to the qualitative research paradigm, this is the only way in which realistic information about sensitive issues can be gained. In palliative-care research, vulnerability for the research participant can often arise because people involved in the study are approaching death. This can create something of emotional tension or communication awkwardness, as reported by Cannon (1989: 66): 'it was not uncommon for women to be sick during the interview and most cried at some time during the series of interviews'. In the same study, one participant, Hilary, said: 'I think I can talk about this today. I haven't got that feeling of distress yet. But when I feel it coming on I'll stop' (1989: 66). In these situations, both the participant and the researcher have to cope with their own emotions and identity crises.

Awkward situations surrounding communication arise when letters are sent, or telephone contact initiated to people who have died. Lindop and Cannon (2001) make reference to a telephone call made to one woman with breast cancer, only to discover that she had died between the return of a consent form and the telephone contact arrangements for the interview. Researchers need enormous skill and empathy to cope with, for example, the partner of the woman who answers the telephone and says that his partner has died.

An equivalent situation occurs when a questionnaire is inadvertently sent to someone who has died. Hospital records, although usually accurate, cannot keep abreast of death which has not yet been recorded, so these kinds of sensitive issue are always waiting for the researcher. However, some of these situations can be reframed as a positive experience, as Lee (1995: 21) notes: 'research on sensitive topics often reveals a desire by research participants for catharsis rather than sanctuary'. Indeed, it should be the rule — always, in all situations, with due consideration to the present and past experiences of the participant — for the researchers of sensitive issues to negotiate a way through the research process.

Research and the consumer experience

In many ways, participants of research represent the consumer experience in that the research should be undertaken to enable a better understanding of the patient's situation so that people in the same predicament in future can be helped more effectively. Lindop and Cannon (2001) adopted a consumer-orientated approach when assessing the needs of women in North Staffordshire, UK, who had diagnoses of breast cancer. They discovered that women's needs related to issues such as wanting information, support from their partner, family and friends, as well as needs associated with body image and sexuality. These needs varied depending on their age and their surgical and medical treatment regimes. If the consumer's perspective of service or care is important, then this should include the views of people with learning disability who are now considered to be ordinary members of the community. Society may have closed the large institutions but this has not stopped the disenfranchisement of this often-vulnerable group.

Research then, if consumer-orientated, is concerned with the patient's experience, just as care should be. On many occasions, research and care become one process. Research that asks patients to comment on their care can be problematic because patients may be reluctant to be critical, feeling that complaints are a sign of ingratitude. Other problems arise when the patient's experience becomes the central focus of the research through such methods as phenomenology. Communicating with patients who are in the palliative stages of their illness during the research process can be inadvertently associated with breaking bad news in that a patient exploring their feelings through, for example, an interview could discover some disturbing information that may previously have been denied. It can be difficult to ask patients about their diagnosis or prognosis if, for instance, they do not know, or do not wish to know, about their illness.

This is an important consideration where someone does not wish to know. The research of Greer (1991) illustrates that denial can be a positive factor in people coping with their illness. The mechanism of denial, according to Greer, is not the psychological defence mechanism previously mentioned and originally described by Freud — but one where the patient accommodates the news but states that they just wish to get on with their lives. Such sensitive points need to be considered because research can be inextricably entwined with care.

A consumer perspective is also important in relation to the family and loved ones, especially in the context of palliative-care research. Indeed, it is often felt more feasible to collect information from relatives of the patient following the patient's death, rather than attempt to intrude into someone's last hours of life. This can overcome the problem of having an unrepresentative sample of patients in a study because many die before they can be interviewed. Using relatives in a study enables a representative sample to be drawn. However, there are dangers in treating relatives' views as if they accurately represent those of the patient. Muncie *et al* (1997), who interviewed 315 competent people over the age of sixty-five as well as individuals who would become their charges if this became necessary, provide an instance of this. The study found that proxies' decisions for their charges were significantly related to the proxies' decision for themselves. Another example is provided by Curtis and Fernester (1989) who found that patients gave pain significantly lower ratings than did their relatives. Interviewing people after the death of a loved one also presents the problem that bereaved relatives' views will be influenced by bereavement and may differ from their views before the patient's death.

Research and learning disability

The question was raised earlier about whether or not people who are disadvantaged, vulnerable or powerless should be involved in research. As White and Barnitt (2000) point out, people with a learning disability fulfill all three criteria. So, the logical question is — should people with a learning disability be involved in research?

The answer is complex, not least of all because people with a learning disability have in the past been exploited as subjects without their consent (by the Nazis, for example). However, there are more recent examples cited in the work of Freedman (2001: 131): the Willowbrook State School experiment in the USA in the 1950s to 1970s, for example, in which children with 'mental retardation' were injected with strains of the hepatitis virus in order to study the progress of the disease; or the experiments between 1944 and 1974 whereby residents of two Massachusetts institutions for people with 'mental retardation' were given minute tracer doses of radiation in breakfast cereal to study mineral absorption in the human body. In both cases, parents gave their consent to the study, but were not informed of the risks.

Ethical considerations are paramount when considering research that involves those who have a learning disability. Informed consent is critical when conducting any research and especially so among prospective participants with a learning disability. Informed consent involves providing clear information, allowing time for questions and time to reflect. However, people with learning disabilities may find it difficult to understand information — and to say no. According to Freeman (2001), understanding has three elements:

- capacity
- voluntarism
- information.

Capacity and voluntarism

Capacity refers to the ability to acquire knowledge, including the ability to express choices and engage in a rational process of making decisions. Voluntarism implies a freedom to exercise choice without being coerced or without any kind of threat, inducement or undue influence. Information involves the ability to grasp facts, especially related to a request to participate in a research project and to appreciate how the research applies to the person's life. Eldridge (2003: 67), citing Beauchamp and Childress, points out that the inequality in knowledge and vulnerability between investigators and subjects has the potential to lead to relationships that are exploitative. Being able to say no is an important consideration, not only in the context of being able to assess whether or not someone's intention is professional, but also in a broader social context. This social context is important since many people with learning disabilities have lived in institutions, often for most of their lives, and now find themselves in a more community-orientated setting. While this change may be more socially desirable, many institutional conditioning processes can remain. For example, being conditioned to meal times; going to bed and rising at particular times; having a bath when directed to; being instructed what to wear and where to go. This institutional conditioning from the past (and still perhaps prevailing at present) can influence the individual's ability to say no.

According to Kerr *et al* (1996), 50% of people with a learning disability present with communication impairment, which can involve hearing, speech and language, all of which can affect cognitive functioning. Many, including Read (2003), rightly argue that good communication is the key to effective palliative care. It is also the key to good research where sensitive issues prevail. Apart from the communication barriers identified, there are many other barriers such as past prejudices related to assumptions that people with learning disabilities need less social consideration. Many such attitudes arose from institutionalisation where it was considered correct to apply block treatment to learning-disability inmates and to dissolve their identity into institutionalised regimes.

Information

However, it can be argued that many professionals simply do not have either the skills or the confidence to communicate effectively with learning-disability people because other community professionals have replaced the carers who were trained and qualified nurses in the field of learning disabilities. An example of this is that nurses trained in the general nursing field, who lack the communication expertise needed to communicate well with this client group, rely on others for their understanding of people with learning disabilities (Lindop and Read, 2000). Ironically, transferring people with learning disabilities from institutional to community settings has to some extent improved social adjustment but deprived them of communication expertise.

Heightened communication skills are necessary in all three areas: learning disabilities, palliative care and research. At a basic level, observing and understanding the characteristic behaviour of people with learning disabilities is a natural starting point. This is especially true in relation to people with a profound disability who are unable to make their feelings known through the normal channels of verbal and non-verbal communication. Changes in normal patterns of behaviour are often the first sign of physical or emotional disturbances. These changes could range from someone being reasonably happy or comfortable to becoming either withdrawn or aggressive. There may be minor signs, such as changes in a pattern of obsessional behaviour, holding the head or rubbing the body. Indeed, such changes may be the first sign of such symptoms as pain.

If people with learning disabilities have less complex needs and they have some ability to communicate, there are several creative strategies of working. Read (1999) applied a number of these when exploring the bereavement-counselling process among people with learning disabilities. A simple approach, according to Read, is directly to alter the techniques that would be used with clients without a learning disability of the same age. This could involve simply adjusting the use of language by making concepts more concrete. Another way could be to reduce the number of ideas discussed at any one time. It might also be possible to involve the person more in the communication process by means of setting simple homework tasks — for instance, how someone felt at the time of loss. This could then be expanded on during the next meeting.

Stories that describe someone else who appears to be in the same predicament or suffering the same symptoms are also useful in that the person can sometimes be encouraged to finish the story. Picture work is especially important in such things as symptom recognition. It is much easier for someone who cannot speak or who has a limited vocabulary to point to a part of the body on a picture to indicate an area of pain. This is also true of pictures that describe the pain, for example whether it is stabbing or burning. Scenarios shown as a sequence of pictures or presented as a story provide another valuable approach to effective communication. Read (2003: 102) outlines an imaginative approach to exploring issues around bereavement and consent to bereavement counselling research. Concept-related cue cards are presented, such as the picture of a coffin and people with flowers around a grave, to clarify understanding, explore questions or queries and help individuals explore their feelings associated with the bereavement experience. Sign language is also a valuable tool for the researcher communicating with learning-disability people.

Science vs sensitivity

Reflecting on the appropriateness of different research methods in palliative care, and their application to people with learning disabilities, it is difficult to avoid the debate about science versus sensitivity. It could be argued that mainstream medicine has lost its sensitivity and is obsessed with scientific proof as its way forward, whether this is related to surgical techniques or clinical trials. Indeed, much of the care concept is also associated with the science of 'doing things to people'. While physical aspects of care are obviously important, they are only one part of the whole. Indeed, while palliative care recognises the importance of physical care, it equally identifies the significance of the other characteristics that go to make up the whole person. This point is made by the World Health Organisation (WHO) (1990) cited by Kinghorn and Gamlin (2001: 7): 'control of pain, of other symptoms, and of psychological, social and spiritual problems is paramount'.

The difficulty associated with symptom management (including pain) is widely known by those working in the field of palliative care. The guiding rule for this was set with the now well-known definition by Mcaffery (1999: 17): 'pain is whatever the experiencing person says it is, existing whenever he says it does'. But what of people with a learning disability with palliative care needs who are experiencing pain and other symptoms when they have problems communicating their experience? This is a real challenge, and requires a high level of communication of the kind previously discussed. Furthermore, given that palliative care resides in the domain of the physician and specialist palliative care team, what happens to those in the community who have a learning disability as well as palliative care needs? It is evident that not enough education and training goes into the preparation of professionals in relation to dealing with these unique types of problems.

Spirituality and learning disability

Symptom management is a challenge, but there are other challenges — for instance, spiritual care. Dyson *et al* (1997) argue that a central component of spirituality is the search for meaning. If an individual is unable to find meaning, all domains of life may be affected, causing spiritual distress. The search for meaning to life is not the privilege of those of us considered to be complete in mind and body, but also of those who have a learning disability as well. Meaning can be embodied in, as Dyson *et al* (1997) suggest, a belief in either God, self or others. One of the central problems hindering the definition of spirituality is its relationship with religion. Indeed, Dyson *et al* (1997: 1185), quoting the work of Steiger and Lipson, argue that religion is a social institution in which a group of people participate, rather than an individual search for meaning. A belief in God, although an abstract concept, could be adopted by learning-disability people in the more concrete form of the 'good father' (an imaginary father figure who watches over us). After all, it can be said that we still live in a paternalistic society.

If we accept that spirituality can be related to God, self or others, we would be able to embrace the holistic concept within this. Indeed, the separation into physical, social, psychological and spiritual in itself contradicts the notion of the whole person by taking a systems approach in an attempt to understand spirituality. If there is for some people a social spirituality, it explains the acute responses that can result from such things as social isolation and loss. Serious illness is often accompanied by both these experiences, and can result in spiritual distress. A terminal illness can rob someone of their sense of wholeness. People with learning disabilities are probably more vulnerable to spiritual distress in a social context than other members of society. Ageing parents or other relatives at home care for many people with learning disabilities. When these carers die, this commonly results in a sense of social isolation and bereavement when the person with a learning disability is forced to experience alternative care.

Some people's spirituality comes from their reliance on self and the capacity for individual survival. Some people can find peace in themselves through the development of their own coping strategies, which bring to them a sense of spiritual ease. This can be the case in the palliative-care situation where someone feels that they can die in peace having organised their affairs and left all things in place as they would wish. The concept of a spiritual self is probably the most complex of the three aspects of spirituality, but it is in this domain that complementary therapy seems to reside, and may provide the most relevant explanation of how people can achieve an inner sense of peace.

Complementary therapies

Complementary therapies of a physical kind have been used among children who have learning disabilities. For example, the sunflower method includes nutritional assessment and supplementation, osteopathic evaluation and neurolinguistic programming (Bull, 2002). However, complementary therapies can interconnect with the social and religious dimensions of spirituality. Kohn (1999) states that the most widely used touch therapies are aromatherapy, reflexology and massage. As Autton (1996: 121) notes, no symbol can be as powerful as a gesture of friendship and no action as meaningful as a dimension of commitment and trust. Hegarty and Gale (1996) show the value of touch as a therapeutic medium for people with challenging behaviours. They present a case study of Ms K whose long-standing challenging and disturbed behaviour was modified through the use of a simple form of massage. Ms K enjoyed this and it was used as a means for communicating positive regard, which led to Ms K becoming more sociable. Most of the complementary therapies that can be used without requiring a reasonable level of cognitive ability — for example, snoezelen, which consists of exposure to relaxing visual, tactile and auditory stimulation (Haggar and Hutchinson, 1991) — could be valuably applied to people with learning disabilities and those with palliative-care needs of spiritual comfort.

Conclusion

In this chapter, I have attempted to link the main research methodologies with sensitive research issues and palliative care. It has also been argued that people with learning disabilities are neglected where palliative care needs are concerned, and remain a disenfranchised group despite being accommodated in the community as opposed to large institutions. Research should be pursued among people with a learning disability to ascertain their views as consumers in general and of health services in particular. Research methods associated with sensitive research among people with learning disabilities need to be carefully selected so as to be ethically appropriate and unobtrusive; this would enable the palliative care needs of learning-disabled people to be detected more clearly. Better and wider education and training of professionals should be undertaken to rectify the deficit of knowledge about learning disabilities and especially communication. This would improve symptom management and, in particular, pain; it would also assist professionals in making relevant assessment of palliative-care needs. The holistic needs of people with learning disability should be considered, especially their spiritual needs. The potential for complementary therapy as an aspect of holistic care should be further explored among this client group.

References

Autton N (1996) The use of touch in palliative care. *Eur J Palliat Care* 3(3): 121–4

Addington-Hall JM, MacDonald LD, Anderson HR, Chamberlain J, Freeing P, Bland JM,

Raferty J (1992) Randomised controlled trial of effects of co-ordinating care for terminally ill cancer patients. *BMJ* **305**: 1317–21

Atkinson D (1988) Research interviews with people with mental handicaps. *Mental Handicap Res* **1**(1): 75–90

Bull L (2002) Parents' use of complementary medicine with their children who have learning difficulties: the case of the sunflower method. *Early Child Dev Care* **172**(3): 247–57

Cannon S (1989) Social research in stressful settings: difficulties for the sociologist studying the treatment of breast cancer. *Sociol Health Illn* **11**(1): 62–77

Curtis AE, Fernester J (1989) Quality of life of oncology hospice patients. In: Field D, Clark D, Corner J, Davis C (2001) *Researching Palliative Care*. Open University Press, Buckingham

Dyson J, Cobb M, Forman D (1997) The meaning of spirituality. *J Adv Nurs* **26**: 1183–8

Eldridge P (2003) Ethics and research involving people with learning disabilities. In: Markwick A, Parrish A (2003) *Learning Disabilities: Themes and Perspectives*. Elsevier Health Science, Philadelphia

Freedman RI (2001) Ethical challenges in the conduct of research involving persons with mental retardation. *Ment Retard* **39**(2): 130141

Greer S (1991) Psychological response to cancer and survival. *Psychol Med* **21**: 43–9

Haggard LE, Hutchinson RB (1991) Snoezelen: an approach to the provision of a leisure resource for people with profound and multiple handicaps. *Ment Handicap* **19**: 51–5

Hegarty JR, Gale E (1996) Touch as a therapeutic medium for people with challenging behaviours. *Br J Learn Disabil* **24**: 26–32

Kerr M, Fraser W, Felce D (1996) Primary health care needs for people with a learning disability. In: Markwick A, Parrish A (2003) *Learning Disabilities: Themes and Perspectives*. Elsevier Health Science, Philadelphia

Kohn M (1999) *Complementary Therapies in Cancer Care*. Macmillan Cancer Relief, London

Lindop E, Read S (2000) District nurses' needs: palliative care for people with learning disabilities. *Int J Palliat Nurs* **6**(3): 117–22

Lindop E, Cannon S (2001) Experiences of women with a diagnosis of breast cancer: a clinical pathway approach. *Eur J Oncol Nurs* **5**(2): 91–9

Lee RM (1995) *Doing Research on Sensitive Topics*. Sage Publications, London

McCaffery M, Pasero C (1999) *Pain*. 2nd ed. Mosby, London

Muncie HL, Magaziner J, Hebel JR, Warren JW (1997) Proxies' decisions about clinical research participation for their charges. *J Am Soc Geriatr Dent* **45**: 929–33

McCarthy M (1998) Interviewing people with learning disabilities about sensitive topics: a discussion of ethical issues. *Br J Learn Disabil* **26**: 140–5

Owen S (2001) The practical, methodological and ethical dilemmas of conducting focus groups with vulnerable clients. *J Adv Nurs* **36**(5): 652–8

Read S (1999) Creative ways of working when exploring the bereavement counselling process. In: Blackman N, Sinason V (1999) *Living with Loss*. Pavilion Publishing, Brighton

Read S (2003) Bereavement and loss. In: Markwick A, Parrish A (2003) *Learning Disabilities:*

Themes and Perspectives. Elsevier Health Science, Philadelphia

Townsend J, Frank AO, Fermont D, Dyer S, Karren O, Walgrove A, Piper M (1990) Terminal cancer care and patients' preference for place of death: a prospective study. *BMJ* **301**: 415–17

White E, Barnitt R (2000) Empowered or discouraged? A study of people with learning disabilities and their experience of engaging in intimate relationships. *Br J Occup Therap* **63**(6): 170–6

World Health Organisation (WHO) (1990) Cancer, pain relief and palliative care. In: Kinghorn S, Gamlin R (2001) *Palliative Nursing: Bringing Comfort and Hope*. Bailliere Tindall, London

INDEX